When Life is a Bit Meh, You Need Energy!

Radical New Ways to Revitalize and Recharge Your Life

Tony Wrighton

LEGAL & DISCLAIMER

Serious, but necessary. The information contained in this book is not designed to replace or take the place of any form of medicine or professional medical advice. The information in this book has been provided for educational and entertainment purposes only.

The information contained in this book has been compiled from sources deemed reliable, and it is accurate to the best of the Author's knowledge; however, the Author cannot guarantee its accuracy and validity and cannot be held liable for any errors or omissions. You must consult your doctor or get professional medical advice before using any suggested remedies, techniques, or information in this book.

Upon using the information contained in this book, you agree to hold harmless the Author, and Publisher, from and against any damages, costs, and expenses, including any legal fees potentially resulting from the application of any of the information provided by this guide. This disclaimer applies to any damages or injury caused by the use and application, whether directly or indirectly, of any advice or information presented, whether for breach of contract, tort, negligence, personal injury, criminal intent, or under any other cause of action. You agree to accept all risks of using the information presented inside this book. You need to consult a professional medical practitioner in order to ensure you are both healthy enough and able to make use of this information. Legal bit over. Let's re-energize.

Manage your meh sections

EXERCISE

COLD — 58

MIND — 74

What to expect

Feeling low energy or depleted? No problem! Strap in for a world first: a fusion of Neuro-Linguistic Programming (NLP) and Biohacking. It's a unique meh-busting approach to living with more energy. Here's what you can expect in this book.

■ **NATURE:** We start by soaking up the energizing power of the natural world. Then we delve into the weird and wonderful world of primal accessories to reconnect and feel more alive.

■ **EXERCISE:** We take a look at the new, radical workouts which can boost our mood, circulation, brain and body. With these exercise techniques, we can invigorate our day and sleep better at night—win-win.

■ **COLD:** As the temperature plummets, the levels of happy chemicals increase in our brain. We investigate all the different ways in which cold can help you to maintain a natural state of mind and body, overcome fear and feel energized.

■ **MIND:** Now it's time to switch on our brain. We explore radical ways to harness our brainwaves, use neurofeedback, access deeper states and unleash our potential. Prepare to fizz with energy.

■ **FUEL:** Hey, snaccidents happen! Don't worry about it. In this section, we start to follow some fuel rules, fuel timings, and specific fuel boosters (supplements) for mood, memory, immunity and energy.

■ **ALCOHOL:** We devote a whole section to that most noble of causes: managing our hangovers. It's time to stay energized while drinking (responsibly, of course).

■ **HOME:** If you want more energy, you need to tackle "meh" on the home front. We go non-toxic, low-EMF, super-natural and clutter-free. We reduce screentime (don't worry - only a bit). And guess what: our energy goes through the roof.

■ **SLEEP:** You can't have energy without rest. We learn how to increase melatonin and REM sleep, avoid "blue light" in the evening, get a longer, deeper rest, and banish sleep FOMO (yep, that's a thing.)

Once you've explored the hundreds of methods (or meh-thods) in the above sections, it is time for...

■ **MEH-TRICS:** This is where the magic happens. In this final section, we bring together everything we've learned in order to ensure you're choosing the methods that work best for you. We collect stats on HRV, sleep, diet, health, and even DNA to create our own unique energy template.

And if you want even more information to continue your energy education, check out...

■ The **MEH DIRECTORY.** Here, you'll find a comprehensive, up-to-date list of products, services, books and practices to re-energize and recharge.

Introduction

meh

/me/

INFORMAL
exclamation: **meh**

1 expressing a lack of interest or enthusiasm; "Meh, I'm not impressed so far."

ADJECTIVE
adjective: **meh**

1 unenthusiastic; apathetic. "Everyone else I talked to was kind of meh."

Do you find yourself having "meh moments"? Are times tough? Do you feel a bit low energy?

You are not alone.

There's an explosion in people feeling more anxious and less satisfied. We spend more of our lives staring at screens and less time staring into the eyes of actual humans than ever before. We have more to worry about and less to energize us. We are constantly busy. We're permanently wired and a bit tired.

Pandemics, political turmoil and toilet roll shortages have all contributed towards this gnawing fatigue. Alongside these deep-seated worries about money, health and family, it sometimes feels as though our lives have shrunk a little and lost some of their sparkle. There's also the loneliness that comes from less human contact. Let's be honest, Zoom doesn't count.

We just feel a bit "meh", and we can't shake it off.

It is, you might say, a meh-pidemic.

My Personal Meh

Unfortunately, I have deep personal experience of meh. Mine got really bad. And despite having written three self-improvement books, I just couldn't shake it off.

It appeared in the most unexpected location. I woke up to shafts of bright sunlight coming through the window of my log cabin. I was at a world-famous retreat called "The Farm" in the Philippines. The Farm is one of the top health and wellness destinations in the world, and you can pick from pool, garden, or jungle-style accommodation. It was an epic place.

I'd chosen the jungle option and, as I lay in bed, I had nothing more to worry about than listening to the exotic sounds of the birds tweeting outside the window, stumbling through the tree canopy to my fancy breakfast, and choosing between yoga or Pilates later that day. This was seven years ago: a much-needed holiday to escape from the stresses of working life in London.

As I swung one leg out of bed, I noticed something strange. I had the bright red stripe of a rash up one leg. I felt a twinge of unease. It was quite a dark red. Not the kind of color you want to see on your leg. I swung the other leg out—all fine on that side. *It's just one of those weird things that comes and goes,* I told myself. I stood up and noticed for the first time that I had an unusual headache. It was strange, different from a normal headache: more of a numbness in my forehead. My anxiety started to rise, but I decided to try and continue with my day as normal.

I emerged from the jungle to approach the Alive! Restaurant. (Yes, the restaurant really was called Alive!) I barely noticed the majestic mountains in the distance, nor my "nutrient rich vegan breakfast." I am a good worrier. And, on this occasion, it actually felt like I had something valid to worry about.

I polished off my breakfast and looked down. *Oh shit.* There was a scarlet red stripe on my other leg now, too. Not a particularly good look in shorts. I wasn't feeling very "Alive!" Time to escape the restaurant.

By the evening, the rash had spread to my torso. I went to see a local doctor. He was sure I had some kind of virus. I started to try and figure out what the issue might be and, after a number of hours consulting with Dr. Google, I'd pretty much self-diagnosed every major communicable disease. The next day the rash had spread to my chest and the numbing headaches had increased. My dream holiday was in tatters. On the flight home, I anxiously ruminated on what was going on with my face and body.

Back in London, I started to feel a bit better. The rash gradually faded. The headaches were still there, but I found I could live with them. I was feeling almost normal. *Weird.* In a jet-lagged haze, I even considered flying back out to The Farm. It was a completely impractical idea to fly across nine time zones once again, especially when I was due back at my job a few days later. But I was tired, wired, and gutted about my holiday. I wasn't thinking straight. In any case, my bank balance was at zero after the emergency flight home, so the decision was made for me. I eased myself back into my work once again, unaware that my problems had only just started.

As well as being an author, I get to talk about and watch sport on TV for a living. It's a very enjoyable job which requires lots of energy and focus. When that energy isn't there, everybody notices—the producers, directors, crew and, of course, the viewers watching at home. I'd always thrived in that environment of TV urgency, but I started to find the work arduous. The headaches came back, along with a deep lethargy. My tropical illness clearly hadn't gone away. I started to wonder how I could confidently present to the world when I felt so depleted. I reluctantly asked for two days off to recuperate.

That "couple of days off" would turn into three months in bed.

Most of that time was spent staring at the ceiling, feeling nauseous and depressed, and wondering if I'd ever get back to full health. The few times I emerged from the house were to visit neurologists, immunologists, and other experts. I was obsessed with trying to figure out what was going on. *What did the low energy levels mean? What about the physical pain? Why did I have weird headaches?* I visited a neurologist on five separate occasions and underwent a number of scans. They started to recognize me at the hospital.

The neurologist explained to me that they could tell from my blood count that I'd had a virus. But they weren't sure exactly which one. *Great.* It turns out there are a number of viruses out there in the world that modern medicine hasn't discovered. Many of them create some kind of post-viral symptoms. I empathize with those going through Long Covid post-viral symptoms, as mine ticked a number of those boxes too. Virus: check. Complications: check.

Health and money worries: check. Deprived of human contact and unsure when things would get back to normal: check.

At one of my lowest points, I was lying in bed, aching all over. I felt the pressure on my forehead and wished I had enough energy to go for a ten-minute walk up the street. But I didn't. I decided to make a pledge to myself. If I ever got back to some half-decent level of health, I'd do something useful. I'd use my journalism and NLP skills to start investigating the topic of energy. I wasn't quite sure how, but I knew from (obsessive) googling that there was a high demand for this information. It became clear that there was a whole spectrum of unexplained fatigue symptoms. Sufferers ranged from the very serious chronic cases who couldn't leave the house, to the hundreds of thousands of people who simply felt a bit burnt out: people exhausted by the pressures of work, social life and social media, working parents with barely enough energy to play with their kids at the end of the day, and even students who couldn't escape a cycle of wired and tired. They all had low-level "meh."

A Search for Zest

After three long months, I slowly started to recover. I tentatively started to think about work. My producers were very kind and understanding. They gave me one short presenting slot on air a week that wouldn't tax me too much.

Those short shifts were a struggle though. I would feel anxious and washed out at work. But I started to feel a shaky confidence that my health was returning. After nine months of gently easing myself back into the working world and going back to my regular work pattern, I *still* had symptoms. It was time to properly start my search for the cure to my persistent fatigue.

At this point, I decided to start a podcast and blog called Zestology. It would be a journey. Yes, I used the J-word. It was indeed a journey to recharge and revitalize myself. I wanted to help people, but—honestly—the main reason for this venture was quite selfish. I needed it for me. I wasn't just looking for more vitality, I was also struggling to hold down my job as a TV presenter, and I was desperate to rediscover my mojo. I wanted to get back to "normal."

So off I went on my adventure to find more energy, vitality and motivation. I investigated every wellness hack that promised to deliver the vitality I was looking for. I dove into the burgeoning worlds of biohacking, health tech, supplements and gadgets. I experimented with crazy new health trends and technology designed to boost performance, energy, and everything in between. I devoured the latest science. I tried the decidedly non-scientific stuff too. I was lucky enough to speak to many of the most respected, well-known experts on the planet. I got bolder and started to try ideas that some people called "extreme." Occasionally, my experimentation went wrong. Think of it this way: I made plenty of mistakes, so you don't have to.

So, what happened?

My energy levels started going up, up, up. It was subtle at first and, over time, it was *extraordinary.*

The podcast became modestly successful, featuring some of the biggest worldwide names in health, medicine, science and wellness. These included figures like Dave Asprey, creator of Bulletproof Coffee and "Father of Biohacking", Joe Wicks, the famous Body Coach and all-round nice guy, and relationship expert and NYT bestselling author Esther Perel," Check out www. tonywrighton.com if you'd like to listen to those and other podcasts.

Some key themes began to appear throughout my research and interviews, and those are the themes you'll read about in the book. These became the foundation for my life. It's been quite the project. I'm now happy to say that, through the findings in this book, I can save you seven years of research, thousands of notes and observations, and multiple experiments that went wrong, and present you with an energy template that will work for you—forever.

The Unique Approach of NLP+B

This book merges my two areas of expertise: the psychological approach of Neuro-Linguistic Programming (NLP) and the exciting new world of Biohacking. 'NLP+B,' if you like.

I started training in NLP almost 20 years ago. It's a powerful set of techniques focusing on how people communicate with themselves and others. We can use NLP to rewire our inner thought processes, and ensure the changes we make are for keeps. I have trained to the very highest level in these skills (Master Practitioner and Trainer). My three NLP-related books have so far been translated into twelve languages, including Chinese, Spanish, Japanese, Turkish, Dutch and Croatian.

As I continued on my journey, I started to have significant personal energy wins when I combined the skills of NLP with a newer concept known as biohacking.

Biohacking uses natural—often forgotten—secrets to optimize your energy, health and performance. When nature isn't available, then it uses radical tech to help. My friend and well-known biohacker Tim Gray says it's about "using technology to mimic a natural environment in an unnatural world."

I've discovered that combining the power of NLP and Biohacking (NLP+B) creates a potent series of self-improvement techniques. The biohacking helps us create instant and powerful energy shifts. Adding in some simple NLP helps them to stick.

The Law of Requisite Variety

I want to introduce an NLP principle straight away. It'll serve you well as you strive to get the most out of this book. "The Law of Requisite Variety" basically says:

"The more variety you can introduce into your life, the more you can adjust and operate at your best."

This is a law well worth respecting on your energy quest. It means you should be as open-minded and flexible as possible. It tells us that when we're doing something that isn't working, we should try something else. That's why there is a rich selection of methods for re-energizing in this book.

You'll find everything from ancient, forgotten practices, to supplements, apps, wearable health tech and deep psychological work. Each of them will help you to recharge and revitalize. Most are free or have a free option available. Some of these methodologies will cost money—a few are expensive. Unfortunately, sometimes the latest health solutions cost big bucks, but I believe that these revitalizing techniques should be accessible to everyone. Therefore, I will always provide you with a cheaper alternative where possible. With the help of this book, my hope is that you will find the techniques that work best for *you,* your lifestyle, and your budget. And that this will lead you along your path to a long, happy, energized life.

The key is to try lots of them. Not all of them will resonate with you, but The Law of Requisite Variety says that the more you sample different techniques, the more you can effectively re-energize. As you approach them with an open mind, you may be surprised at how well they work.

Here's how to read this book:

1. Start to get acquainted with the methods for re-energizing yourself. Read them cover to cover, or else feel free to dip in and out of the ones that appeal to you.

2. In the final MEH-TRICS section, we investigate the techniques that make you feel most energized, and we compile more data.

3. You end up with your own unique template for operating at your best.

If You Can Measure It, You Can Change It

Let's talk a bit more about metrics or, as I call them in this book, meh-trics. As I started to recover from my tropical virus, I threw myself into trying anything and everything that might give me some extra sparkle. Some techniques had an instant impact. I started feeling a little bit better. The dietary and lifestyle tweaks were starting to invigorate me, but I didn't know which ones. *Was it the extra helping of veggies? Was it that workout? Or perhaps the extra hour of sleep helped?* I never quite knew what was effective and what wasn't. I didn't have the evidence yet.

Another guiding principle in NLP is an obsessive focus on "doing what works'", whatever that might be. So, I started looking for energizing trends as I went. *Did supplements mean a better night's sleep? Did mindfulness improve my mood? Which of these changes was giving me a boost?* I started to discover what was firing me up so I could do more of it.

Gathering metrics is all about figuring out how you know when you feel meh, and what shifts it. That makes me your guide, not your guru. The true indicator of what works for you will be your metrics. More recently, these analysis techniques have become known as "self-tracking" or the "Quantified Self".

You will reclaim your vitality by asking yourself some key questions in order to identify what works, and I'll guide you through the process. These are examples of the sort of questions you might ask.

- After meditating every day this week, did your stress levels improve compared to last week?

- Have you been sleeping better since you started taking magnesium supplements?

- Do you feel rubbish when you sit on the sofa for ten hours scrolling on Facebook? (Hint: probably.)

To measure our meh level and turn it into something more positive, we ask these questions and then make a note of the answers. In other words, we collect data. Trust me: this is actually more exciting than it sounds, even if you're not convinced right now.

Start trying the techniques in this book right away. Then, when you suspect something is giving you a little jolt of vitality, turn to the MEH-TRICS section. Technology will provide you with interesting, and dare I say it, even fun ways to collect and analyze some evidence. My pledge is that it'll never take more than one minute to collect all your data for the day. When you start collecting your diary metrics, you start to achieve "self-knowledge through numbers"—definitive proof on what energizes you.

"What's measured, improves." Legendary productivity guru, Peter Drucker, said that 40 years ago:

And that includes your meh.

Finally, look out for scientific references and fact-checks throughout. While it is important to me that I share my own story and experience, it is even more important to show how each of these methods is supported by science. Sometimes there is rigorous research, and I've included it. In other instances, something seems to work despite a lack of randomized double-blind controlled studies. I'll be honest about it when that is the case.

This book is an exploration of the radical new ways you can activate deep levels of vitality. The Law of Requisite Variety says you should try as many of them as possible, and then start to make small, incremental changes in your life.

Remember: when life is a bit rubbish, things won't necessarily turn around overnight. But by reading on, you can start to feel significantly more energized, and more quickly than you might expect.

Chapter One

Nature

"

At some point in life, the world's beauty becomes enough.

TONI MORRISON

"

Why this theme?

In our first section, we are going to soak up the energizing power of the natural world. Being in nature can help with anxiety, depression, anger and fatigue (1). Health benefits can include a reduction in blood pressure, heart rate, and stress hormones, and potential preventive effects on cancers (2). That all adds up to a big reduction in meh. Nature makes us feel better. We instinctively know this, and the research confirms it.

So why don't we gravitate towards nature more often?

Is it perhaps because of some of these contradictions?

- We want to feel the pull of nature, but we don't always have time to go to a forest.

- We want to love the great outdoors, but we don't want to give up our screens.

- We want to get closer to the natural world, but we still want to be able to pick up our favorite fancy latte from the local coffee shop on the way, served just the way we like it.

The key is to find ways to embrace our natural state in a decidedly unnatural world.

What can you expect in this section?

We're about to get a little bit less domesticated. We're going to reconnect with our wild, natural side, without having to go camping in the woods for five days.

First we'll explore some forgotten primal ways of living, They're easily applicable to our own lives. Then we'll tap into decidedly technological hacks that help us plug into a natural state. And we'll make use of the weird and wonderful world of primal accessories to reconnect and make us feel more alive.

Let's start by taking some inspiration from great creative minds.

FOREST BATHING: EVERYTHING THAT MAKES LIFE WORTH LIVING COMES THROUGH THE SENSES

As I write this, I'm listening to Gustav Mahler's Symphony No. 5 in C-Sharp Minor. The great man first made his name as a conductor , and as he matured, then became a great composer. Much of his creative work was written in the woods in Southern Austria at a tiny little "composing cottage." His routine was extremely strict. He would wake early, and immediately take himself off to his stone hut in the forest. This was a tiny little dwelling under a canopy of trees. His mornings would consist of woodland solitude. The dappled sunlight would filter through the open door as he ate his modest breakfast alone on a bench.

After his morning's music-making was over, he would take multiple dips in the local lake. Then, he would dry off in the sun and dip in once again. There would be a light lunch. And then long invigorating walks in the afternoon.

Actually, Mahler was at times a grumpy so-and-so. Apparently he "couldn't bear to see anyone" before he started work and his wife was under orders to bribe the neighbors with opera tickets to stop their dogs from barking and disturbing poor Gustav. But he loved the forest, and his great body of work is evidence of its inspiration.

You might say Mahler used Forest Bathing for inspiration. This is now an "in" term for getting outside, but has been acknowledged for many years by many cultures for its rejuvenating power. The Japanese call it Shinrin-yoku. This translates as spending time in a forest and soaking up the sights, sounds and smells of the great outdoors to revive body and soul. That's all. Just doing this is proven to lift your mood.

Admittedly, Forest Bathing does sound a bit pretentious, but here's the thing: it doesn't actually have to be done in a forest.

Consider the word "forest" to be a metaphor. Go anywhere that isn't indoors. Soak up the sights, sounds and smells of nature in your local park. Hug a tree on your street. Bathe in the back garden. The science shows you'll feel less meh.

The challenging bit is being present in nature. It's soaking it up. That's where the meditative side of Neuro-Linguistic Programming can help. NLP is based on how we use our senses to gather information and experience the world. Often, we favor one sense and we miss much of what is going on. Learning to switch on the senses—especially in nature—is one of the most important ways we can re-energize. As NLP author Joseph O'Connor says,

"Joy, pleasure, understanding and keenness of thought, everything that makes life worth living comes through the senses."

If you find your mind wandering, take inspiration from this NLP routine. I do it regularly to relax while in nature.

- Focus on three things you can see. Concentrate on each one. Notice colors, shade, light and distance.

- Notice three things you can hear. Tune in. Notice volume, pitch and clarity.

- Now focus on three things that you can feel or touch, like the temperature of the air, or the feeling of a wet bum as you sit on a damp log.

- Keep cycling through what you can see, hear, and feel. Can you do it for a few minutes? Sometimes I struggle to focus on this technique for 30 seconds, which just shows me how much I need it in that moment.

- Finish, and notice how much more present and in the moment you are.

Making full use of your visual, auditory and kinesthetic senses is the perfect accompaniment to forest (or garden or park) bathing. You are opening your senses to the things that makes life worth living.

KEEPING IT WALKABLE: ONE OF THE CRUCIAL PLANKS OF LONGEVITY

If you live near a forest, you are probably congratulating yourself right now. And why not? You can pop out for a spot of forest bathing at lunch time. That said, there are major benefits to living in cities too, and it's possible to effectively "reframe" (another NLP technique) where you live.

Research shows that in many cases, living in a city is actually really good for your health. That's because there are many different aspects to living naturally and one of them is to be an active part of the community.

Scientists at Washington State University studied mortality data and found that neighborhood walkability and green spaces are two of the crucial planks of longevity (3). The study followed 145,000 people (which makes it fairly statistically significant), and suggested we want to live somewhere "highly walkable". In other words, cities. This combination of proximity to greenery and easy access to the community is a significant determinant of whether we'll reach age 100. That's obviously relevant to vitality as good health and energy are so interlinked.

So, perhaps you should feel good about living in the city. Maybe you don't have a Mahler-style composing cabin at the end of the garden, but instead you have plenty of parks and friends nearby. Walk as much as you can. Park 15 minutes away when you need to use the car. Set up a local WhatsApp group (or equivalent) to get to know your neighbors.

On our street we lend, recycle, and bake for each other. Every time we step out of the house, there's someone to talk to. It's a ready-made social life and always a good excuse to keep any errands walkable. It's easy to build a community online, but here we are focusing on real-life tribe-building. We want to spend less time looking at pictures of someone else's tea on social media and surround ourselves with ambitious, positive, like-minded people. Ideally, we can walk down the road to go and see our tribe face-to-face.

Prioritize spending time in green spaces nearby, and building your local community. The research suggests you'll be healthier and more energized. You might even live to 100.

GET GROUNDED: ARE YOU JUDGING ME ON MY FLIP-FLOPS?

The earth produces a slight negative charge. When we walk around on it, we can utilize the earth's natural power to encourage a state of healing. The research is compelling. Being connected to the ground can "positively affect morning fatigue levels, daytime energy, and nighttime pain levels" (4). Unfortunately, walking around in your smart leather-soled shoes on the office carpet doesn't count.

That's where the concept known as "earthing" comes in. The earth's energy somehow transfers itself from the ground into the body. This sounds totally wacky, but it's proven by the science. The belief is that grounding to the earth can have a huge impact on your physical and mental state. It works like this.

a) You touch the earth or, if that's not possible

b) You use some kind of equipment to help you.

The equipment to help us with this grounding to the earth is extensive. My first tentative step into this world was with some grounded flip-flops by Pluggz, containing "a proprietary carbon and rubber black plug embedded into the soles which allows for the free flow of electrons from the Earth into our bodies." I have noticed a small energy shift when I wear grounded flip-flops. It's not groundbreaking, but I still wear them because they are comfortable.

There is a dizzying array of mats, sheets, blankets, socks, wristbands and even patches you can invest in to do your grounding. They are like barefoot substitutes. They cleverly conduct the earth's energy to your body, often by connecting to the ground port of an electrical outlet.

You can also go barefoot more. I'm barefoot now, but that's mainly because I'm writing from home. I can walk around my shed in whatever I like. So start off with grounding by going barefoot as much as you can. Then try the tech.

Truthfully, grounding is not my first stop for instant energy, but it does feel good. It feels natural and I know many who swear by it for a connected boost of vitality. And while the tech is almost endless, true grounding is completely free. Just take your shoes off and start walking.

CIRCADIAN RHYTHM: DON'T WEAR SHADES IN THE MORNING

Tapping into our natural circadian rhythm is key to energizing during the day. The best way to do it is with something that is available to all of us: simple daylight. We need as much light as possible in the morning. It'll make us more awake during the day and help us sleep better at night.

So how do we do more of this? Get outside more, obviously, and then something surprising: I met with respected sleep researcher Matthew Walker who told me, "Don't wear shades in the morning."

This is all about resetting your natural body clock. Yes, sunglasses may look cool and shade your eyes, but you need to get all of that daylight into your brain to re-energize and recharge for the day ahead. How we respond to the light-dark cycle is crucial for our health. Light plays a key role in transmitting time of day information to our bodies. It realigns our natural circadian rhythm and even helps alleviate jet lag and night shift sleep problems (5).

I have to prioritize this. Having a job in TV is brilliant, but when we are in the studio it is a very indoor environment. It is the opposite of Mahler's stone hut in the forest that we encountered earlier. I am surrounded by brightly-illuminated screens and no windows. That leads me to place extra emphasis on getting outdoors away from work. I definitely feel more energized when I get plenty of good quality daylight. Here's how easy it is:

- Look out of the window in the morning before you look at your device. (Not something many people do.)

- Prioritize getting loads of morning light—preferably from the sun, but we can't always be picky.

- Get a good morning walk outside without shades, especially if you are then going to be staring at a computer all day.

Remember, more light exposure in the morning leads to better sleep quality at night. So you'll get more energy today and more energy tomorrow too.

INFRARED LIGHT: IS 5 AM TOO EARLY FOR YOU?

Famous American novelist Toni Morrison understood how important morning light is. She described her writing routine as revolving around the sunrise. She would get up about 5am, and sip on her coffee as the sun came up. Being there for the first light of the day was crucial. She said,

"I'm very, very smart in the morning and everything is clear. By noon it's over."

As the day wore on, she said she got "dumber and dumber." She used the power of the sunrise to kickstart her natural energetic rhythm. There's a small problem though: 5 am is just a tiny bit early for me to be setting my alarm clock.

Using near red and infrared light devices is a biohack that can help with that. It certainly fits the "radical alternative" category. Remember, we want to use nature to manage our meh as much as possible. However when nature isn't available (i.e. you don't want to wake up at 5 am, or sunrise is a grey wintery splodge), we can employ such radical alternatives.

So how can an infrared light in your home help?

Red Light delivered at 660nm (the technical light term) is readily absorbed by surface tissues and cells leading to great skin and better healing. Near-Infrared Light delivered at 850nm is invisible to the human eye, and penetrates into deeper tissues. This leads to enhanced recovery, better health, and less inflammation. The idea is that these are just like the wavelengths of light your body needs from sunlight, but without the heat or UV rays that may cause sun damage. And when it comes to managing meh, there are thousands of clinical studies on the power of light therapy (6) to help with inflammation, sleep and energy.

I use infrared lights from Joovv. This is a light company so serious about what they do, they've teamed up with the athletes of the San Francisco 49ers to help their recovery regime. Think burly football players standing in front of lights after games. They believe it helps them heal faster and improve athletic performance. I meditate or work out in front of it in the morning, and the brightness of the light really seems to wake me up, especially in winter. There are plenty of other companies selling good lights too.

So, to recap, here's how you can use light to power up naturally in the morning;

- **Option 1.** Get up to watch the sunrise. This is an awesome option. But if, like me, you don't want to set the alarm for 5 am, then we move to...

- **Option 2.** Use light therapy for many of the same effects.

Either will give you a natural morning boost.

PRIMAL FOOTWEAR: WALKING IN YOUR ANCESTORS' FOOTPRINTS

We've already looked at grounding, and it may not surprise you to know that the average caveman and cavewoman didn't wear shoes. This is your great great great great great great great (plus a lot more "great"s) grandparents we're talking about here, so listen up. They padded around in bare feet, and their toes went exactly where they wanted to go.

As humans started to discover clothes, shoes and fashion, a weird thing happened. We developed a habit for wearing shoes that don't actually fit our feet. We now squish our feet into a container that isn't actually foot-shaped. They're too narrow at the ends. And because we are cramming our feet into shoes that are not shaped correctly, we don't walk the way we were intended to.

Over time, this causes all sorts of postural and structural problems. You could blame your dodgy knees, back and even neck on poor footwear. This is obviously a drain on your energy stores. There are also more obvious issues like bunions, sore feet and toes which also make you feel low. You might even suffer from something I was personally afflicted with for many years—one of the most unattractively titled foot complaints out there—Haglund's deformity. This is an enlargement of the posterosuperior calcaneus, or to you and me, a bony lump on your heel that can become very bothersome.

The solution is to walk like our ancestors did. That doesn't mean walking barefoot to buy some ancient grains in Whole Foods, although you could do that if you really wanted. It means investing in so-called minimalist footwear. These tend to be wide shoes with thin soles, and minimal heel or support. The shoes are designed to give you maximum sensory feedback. They're foot-shaped so your feet can move as intended. Walking around in these shoes feels like walking with no shoes on—and it is a primal feeling. You can feel the difference almost instantly when your feet have been squashed up for so long.

DISCLAI-MEHS

Disclaimer 1. Minimalist footwear, or 'primal shoes' often look a bit... weird. There's no other way of putting it. We are used to elegant looking footwear with narrow toes, and unfortunately that's not the way these shoes are shaped. So, you may not be winning any fashion prizes. Personally, I think all the brands I love (listed in the Meh Directory) look awesome, but then you are not reading this book for my fashion sense.

Disclaimer 2. They are also not the cheapest option. Bringing up a small human and looking at the prices of primal footwear for kids, I may be taking out a second mortgage.

There is a growing number of companies that provide these shoes to help us get back to a natural state. My favorites are Vivo Barefoot (perhaps the most stylish, and the kids' range is epic), LEMS shoes (even wider for my big paddle feet) and Altra trainers (another "zero drop" shoe, which means the sole is the same height as the toe and a little more padded—this cushions the knees a little more).

Primal shoes feel great in the moment and are a long-term health upgrade. They just feel right.

PRIMAL SQUAT: THE BATHROOM ACCESSORY THAT TAKES YOU BACK TO NATURE

It will come as no surprise that our cavewomen and cavemen ancestors did not have lovely porcelain toilets. Squatting, not sitting, was the order of the day for millions of years.

So perhaps our bodies are evolutionarily designed to squat, not sit?

Happily, we don't have to completely rip our bathroom apart to go back to a more primal way of squatting.

My wife gave me the humble Squatty Potty (link in Meh Directory). She's a true romantic. Without going into too much detail, it really works. It helps to elevate your feet while on the toilet. If you don't want to shell out for one, pick some old books you don't read anymore (not this one) and make a couple of delicate toilet piles. In the health world, many hacks can cost a lot. This one doesn't, though, and it's surprising how effective it is.

Why does it help with energy? Well, if I must spell it out: having regular bowel movements is a sign of a healthy digestive system, and it prevents the discomfort of energy drainers like diarrhea and constipation (7). Getting into the right position will help with this regularity.

While we're about it, this is totally unscientific, and backed up with no research, but not checking your phone while you sit on the toilet is probably also a really good idea. Too much? Maybe. You know I'm right though.

VITAMIN D: ESCAPING 50 SHADES OF GREY

As I write this, it's winter. I'm looking out of the garden shed where

I'm writing this book, and the best way to describe the weather is grey. Not epically cold. No biblical storms. Just a lot of grey, stretching as far as the eye can see.

Here in the UK, we endure this greyness, and perhaps even learn to love it. But however much we get outside into nature, we don't get much of "the sunshine vitamin" in the middle of winter. It's called that for a reason. Vitamin D has been found to have a dramatic effect on mood and energy (8). Over 40 patient studies suggest it also mitigates the effects on viruses including COVID-19, reducing infection, severity and mortality (9). Vitamin D supplements are a real staple for many of the natural health experts I've spoken to over the past seven years. They advocate quite a bit more than the recommended daily dose, which is low. Consult with your practitioner before starting any new regime.

Does it give you an extra spark? Yes. When I first started taking it I noticed a significant uptick in mood and vitality. Now, truthfully, it's hard to measure, as I don't want to go without Vitamin D for a month in order to collect more metrics.

Vitamin D is in this section of the book because we get it from nature. But when nature doesn't cooperate and it's 50 Shades of Grey outside your winter, you can supplement. I take 4000–6000 IUs a day of Vitamin D combined with K2 to help absorption. I'm religious about it in winter, and try to get as much of sunshine vitamin in summer as possible.

References

1. Effect of forest bathing (Shinrin-yoku) on human health: A review of the literature—https://pubmed.ncbi.nlm.nih.gov/31210473/
2. A comparative study of the physiological and psychological effects of forest bathing on working-age people with and without depressive tendencies—https://www.ncbi.nlm.nih.gov/pmc/articles/PMC6589172/
3. Environmental Correlates of Reaching a Centenarian Age: Analysis of 144,665 Deaths in Washington State for 2011–2015—https://www.mdpi.com/1660-4601/17/8/2828
4. Earthing: Health Implications of Reconnecting the Human Body to the Earth's Surface Electrons—https://www.ncbi.nlm.nih.gov/pmc/articles/PMC3265077/
5. Human circadian rhythms: physiological and therapeutic relevance of light and melatonin—https://pubmed.ncbi.nlm.nih.gov/17022876/
6. Database of over 1000 light therapy clinical studies—https://joovv.com/pages/clinical-studies
7. Easy ways to stay regular: Improve digestive health by addressing underlying causes of irregularity, as well as fluids, diet, and exercise—https://www.health.harvard.edu/aging/easy-ways-to-stay-regular
8. Vitamin D and Depression: Where is all the Sunshine?—https://www.ncbi.nlm.nih.gov/pmc/articles/PMC2908269/
9. Sixty seconds on . . . vitamin D: Vitamin D Mitigates COVID-19, Say 40+ Patient Studies (listed below)—Yet BAME, Elderly, Care-homers, and Obese are still 'D' deficient, thus at greater COVID-19 risk—WHY?—https://www.bmj.com/content/371/bmj.m3872/rr-5

Meh-busting Nature Reminders...

1

Go forest bathing. Switch on your senses and feel more alive. A garden or park will do if there is no forest nearby.

2

Get good light. Watch the sunrise. Ditch your shades.. Use infrared light when nature isn't playing ball.

3

Go 'primal'. Reconnect with grounding, barefoot shoes, and, er, a squatty potty.

Chapter Two

Exercise

> **There are no FDA-approved medications (nor any in the pipeline) that come close to demonstrating the improvements seen with daily exercise.**

DR. DALE BREDESEN

Why this theme?

We want to boost our mood, circulation, brain and body. Most of us already instinctively know that, if we roll downstairs in our underwear and don't emerge from the house until lunchtime, we can expect to feel meh. And the science proves it.

When it comes to research-led ways to improve our mood and re-energize us, studies keep bringing us back to exercise. They consistently show lots of movement can improve our mental health (1) and health-related quality of life (2, 3). In other words, getting off your ass makes you feel better.

A particularly interesting area to study energy and longevity is people living in blue zones. These are the areas where the lifestyle leads to people living to a particularly ripe old age—including the beautiful Italian island of Sardinia, as well as parts of Okinawa, Greece and Costa Rica. Researchers have found one commonality between life in these places that is particularly significant: lots of moderate exercise throughout the day. Many of the healthiest supercentenarians (those who live to 110 and beyond) "all walked several miles each day throughout their working lives. They never spent much time, if any, seated at desks" (4). Other longevity research suggests Olympians have a "survival advantage" and live an average of 2.8 years longer than the rest of us (5).

So exercise can help us feel better and live longer. Win win.

What can you expect in this section?

We'll take a look at new, radical workouts. With these exercise techniques, we can invigorate our day and sleep better at night. But it's more than just workouts. We've established if we want to feel energized, we need to move. Lots. We're made to do it. The idea is to move as much as possible, all through the day.

For this reason, we are going to build a consistent Getting Off Your Ass Program. Or GOYAP, as it shall be officially known.

Some of these methods of exercise come from the world of biohacking, and explore completely fresh technology, while others have been around centuries.

LOW-LEVEL EXERCISE: BOOST YOUR MOOD AND PRODUCTIVITY

The existentialist philosopher, Søren Kierkegaard, had a GOYAP—though it's highly doubtful he called it that. Ol' Kierkegaard was a famous figure in 1840s Copenhagen. As well as being a philosopher, he was a theologian, poet, social critic, and huge influence on politics, literature and psychology. He was also a WFHer (Work From Homer). So what can we learn from his habits?

He stuck to a particular daily routine to assist his prodigious output. He basically did two things all day. Writing and walking. He'd regularly venture out into the streets of Copenhagen for long walks where he had his best ideas. Sometimes he'd be in such a hurry to get them down on paper that he would have to scramble home. He'd barge through the door and scribble down his thoughts standing up, still wearing his hat (apparently not the thing to do in 1840s Copenhagen). He understood the value of low-level exercise for energy, mood and creativity.

Incidentally, Kierkegaard also had an unusual way of drinking coffee. It was so extraordinary that I feel the need to tell you about it here, even though I don't recommend it. He would take a cup, and fill it to the top with sugar. Then he would drizzle a paltry amount of extremely strong black coffee over it. He would wait until he was satisfied the sugar had dissolved and then sip his syrupy goo.

Nb: Drizzling coffee over a sugar mountain is not one of my energy recommendations.

So here's the plan:

- Incorporate as much movement as possible into your working day

- Do meetings on walks. Take calls while you stroll to the shop.

- Take movement breaks once an hour.

- Tell your boss it'll make you more productive. If they don't buy it, do it anyway.

I find this is an area in which measuring my progress is important for keeping me on track. Anything from a simple step-counter to a sophisticated health watch can help. A number of health trackers now ping us every hour with movement reminders. And they start to provide the evidence for how more exercise positively affects our energy levels. You can head over to the MEH-TRICS section for some ideas on how to do this.

It's notable how many great thinkers like Kierkegaard have used movement as the primary source for their creative output over the years. Fast forward to now and we seem to have forgotten the power of exercise. Your boss might think you are radical if you suggest taking outdoor meetings. Or weird to want a movement break. That's the world we live in: but I encourage you to do it anyway. It's hard to move when you feel tied to your work on a screen. But it's important. As well as some extra get-up-and-go, you might find you are more productive too. Leonardo Da Vinci said this:

"Men of lofty genius when they are doing the least work are most active."

And, of course, the same could be said of women of lofty genius.

Which all reminds me: I've just written this section while locked in my garden shed. I haven't got out for a while. It's time to tap into some Leonardo genius, employ a GOYAP technique and go for a walk.

WFH WORKOUTS: CHANGING YOUR BRAIN WITH EXERCISE

Let's move from light movement to a good, solid workout.

Proper exercise can literally change the composition of your brain and the way it works. Alzheimer's expert Dr. Dale Bredesen noted one particular study in which researchers did brain scans on participants who exercised four days a week for up to an hour. They were split into two groups. One group did stretching, and the others got aerobic exercise on a treadmill. After six months, the results were nothing short of incredible:

Brain imaging showed that those who participated in vigorous aerobic exercise actually had reduced levels of tau, a protein associated with the tangles and neurite retraction of Alzheimer's. Additionally, the aerobic exercisers had better blood flow in the memory and processing centers of their brains as well as measurable improvement in the attention, planning, and organizing abilities referred to as executive function.

Spare a thought for the stretching group. If I ever feel like skipping a workout, I remind myself of this research. It is tangible evidence that strenuous physical exercise is not just good for our short and long-term energy levels, it's also what we're simply meant to do.

In addition, exercise may delay the decline in cognitive function that occurs in individuals who are at risk of or who have Alzheimer's, with aerobic exercise possibly having the strongest effect (6). Radical solutions to age-related disease are exciting, and this research serves as an inspiration to use workouts to live longer and help our brains work better.

So how can you do this at home? Sure, your gym membership might have been downgraded, the fancy ClassPass app has been cancelled, and the occasional trips to the local yoga studio might have dwindled. However proper, clearly-defined exercise is still crucial.

When you are stuck at home and feeling a bit meh, indulge in a radical workout on the living room floor. With the WFH (Working From Home) revolution, there are more new-school workouts springing up every day. In our house, we love these thoroughly modern sites and apps:

▓ Glo (the Rolls Royce of home workouts, lots of options)

▓ P:volve (targeted Pilates-like workouts to improve your core)

▓ The Class (sweaty, genre-defying workouts that challenge mind and body)

▓ Peleton (fun workouts on a standalone app that doesn't involve shelling out big bucks on a bike)

■ Ha'You Fit (where breathwork and fitness meet)

These workouts are not free, but by subscribing to these programs you may even find you save money, as you won't need your gym membership any more.

Remember to combine these full-on exercise routines with lots of moderate exercise to fire up your endorphins and change your mood fast.

AI EXERCISE BIKES: GET FIT IN 40 SECONDS

I travelled to Central London to meet the maker of an "artificial intelligence fitness bike". The makers of the oddly-named CAROL (or CAR.O.L) promise that you can get the same benefits that you would get from a 45-minute jog in two 20-second sprints on their bike. It clearly sounded too good to be true. So, I perhaps rashly agreed to record a podcast while doing their workout. How bad could 40 seconds of exercise be?

When I arrived, Rahul from the company explained how the bike uses artificial intelligence and science to compress a workout into a few seconds. Surprisingly, CAROL is clinically proven to give you the same cardio benefits as a 45-minute jog with just those 40 seconds of hard work. It does this by ensuring you hit max intensity levels and max glycogen depletion in two 20-second sprints. It's a bit like being chased by a tiger. You get a sudden demand for energy. That causes your body to rapidly burn large amounts of sugar stores in the muscles within 5-10 seconds. Then sh!t starts getting real. Your body senses a threat to your survival. Research shows there is a huge surge of those molecules in the body that upgrade you to being fitter, leaner, and healthier (7).

The idea is that this personalized workout will push you harder than any spin class. In just 40 measly little seconds.

Rahul eyed my spindly chicken legs. Perhaps it was becoming evident that I wasn't one of nature's intuitive cyclists. Despite this he cranked the settings up to full. I nervously waited, ready to get chased by the tiger.

Perhaps it wasn't my finest 40 seconds of podcasting. The listeners heard me get—for want of a better expression—absolutely destroyed—in those two 20-second segments. But afterwards, as I walked wobbly-legged back to the tube station, I felt energized. It really did feel like I'd done a 45-minute workout.

I've now got one in my shed here at home. I like the brief, intense push, and the extra time that such a short workout creates.

And I'm promised that I can expect to double my fitness levels too. I'm hoping I'll see the results on my chicken legs...

Owning an AI exercise bike is expensive, so perhaps find one at a local gym, clinic or shop. You only need to use it for ten minutes a couple of times a week to benefit from it.

AI STRENGTH TRAINING: MAGIC BARBELLS

Machines are rapidly changing the ways we work out. That goes for strength training as well as endurance. ARX (Adaptive Resistance Exercise) is a full body workout machine that only takes a few minutes to give you a proper workout. It's strangely exhausting. Building on the artificial intelligence theme, this technology has been created to match the resistance of the user 100% of the time. That means you "get the perfect rep, every time". You'll feel the burn in seconds, not hours.

This type of AI workout helps you build strength more quickly and improve your metabolic conditioning at the same time. The idea behind it is that it's more efficient, and more targeted. You get the results you want more quickly and effectively.

It also works because we can lower a lot more than we can lift. I find it extraordinary that on the "way down" bit of lifting (normally the easier bit), I am straining even more. This is one of the points of difference of ARX. It's said we often "leave a lot of meat on the bone" with normal weights. An AI machine gym won't let you get away with that.

It doesn't matter if you are the world's most dedicated gym jockey, you'll still be straining every sinew. With AI strength training, Mr Universe would be straining just as much as I do. I always walk away feeling the burn, and the next day I always feel sore. It's just like I spent an hour working out, but it only took ten minutes.

You don't need one at home. Find a local gym or clinic with an ARX and try out the magic barbells.

VR WORKOUTS: FUTURISTIC EXERCISE ROUTINES MADE FUN

I have two left feet and cannot dance. But put me into a futuristic Blade Runner-style landscape with a techno soundtrack and a load of flying balls coming at me and I feel I can move like a professional. After 30 minutes, I'm smiling and sweating. If you find workouts boring, Virtual Reality (VR) headsets might be the solution.

VR makes it so much fun to get moving you won't want to stop. I'm quite convinced it's the future of exercise. You put the goggles on, and are magically transported to a radically different reality that encourages you to sweat at the same time. You can choose from workout games like Audio Trip (clever dance exercise workouts with songs from artists like Lady Gaga), Eleven Table Tennis (realistic ping pong), and Synth Riders (futuristic dance game). If you are competitive—even better—you can play against your friends.

I've been using the Oculus Quest 2 for a while and it's insanely addictive. The set-up takes seconds and you don't need to pair it with a TV or computer, just a Facebook account. These exercise options are not substitutes for a workout for me: they're an add-on. VR provides an extra segment of movement in my day as it's just such a blast.

VR is improving so quickly I believe that soon it will be ubiquitous rather than radical. The price is also improving. Oculus Quest 2 starts from $399 (£299), which is what my gym membership costs for four months.

EXERCISE + BREATH: HAVE A QI BREAK

Radical, re-energizing exercise doesn't have to involve working up a full-on sweat, but it can be a little more organized than a simple walk. We've established we want to move as much as possible for our meh-management, and now we move from the distinctly modern to the decidedly ancient.

Qi Gong has long been associated with energy, vitality and banishing meh. Indeed some research shows it results in better general health and vitality compared to other forms of exercise (8). It's a moderate, meditative workout, combining movement, breath, balance and muscle control. That's the idea anyway. I tend to arrange my body into a series of faintly ridiculous positions and hope for the best. These positions often resemble animals or warrior poses and activate energy meridians around the body. It's ancient, but judging by the looks I get when I do it in public, a bit radical too. Without fail, it leaves me feeling revitalized afterwards.

I can often be found practicing my Qi Gong 12 Rivers routine or indulging in some Qi Gong Animal Play in the garden. Once the neighbors see you busting out moves like *Wild Goose Beats Its Wings*, or *Black Tiger Straightens Its Waist*, prepare for them to think you are even stranger than they thought. The strength of the tiger, the balance of the crane... maybe they are right. It does look bizarre, but it is such a powerful energizer.

I made it my mission to try to figure out just what feels so good about QI Gong. My number one theory was that it had to be something to do with the practice's focus on the breath. So, I introduced myself to a number of experts on breathing, including bestselling author and investigative journalist, James Nestor.

He told me that 90% of us—very likely you, me, and almost everyone we know—are breathing incorrectly. This failure is bad for us. It's either causing or aggravating a laundry list of chronic illnesses. Our meh gets worse when we don't breathe right.

He told me when we connect with the breath, we can start to feel energized. And as much as possible, we want to breathe through the nose not the mouth. This will help us to increase circulation, get better sleep, and even stop going to the loo in the middle of the night.

Head to the Meh Directory for some introductory Qi Gong ideas. A light exercise routine that focuses on the breath will invigorate your day and be a useful part of your GOYAP.

MEH-TRICS TO EXPLORE: DESIGNING THE PERFECT WORKOUT

Gathering metrics is a key part of our meh-busting strategy, and measuring your progress after workouts is a powerful area to explore. You can find some particularly interesting correlations that will lead you towards the perfect exercise routine for you. You might want to gather stats in these areas.

■ Use objective metrics from a wearable to provide heart rate, HRV and sleep data.

■ Compare these against subjective measurements like your energy levels, measured out of 10, before and after exercise.

Turn to the MEH-TRICS section for ways to analyze these stats and more inspiration

DO WHATEVER IT TAKES: SOLVING THE GREAT WORKING FROM HOME PROBLEM

Many of us now only need walk from the bedroom to the kitchen table to get to work. But the supercentenarians we looked at earlier do the opposite, all the way through their lives.

■ They walk all day and hardly ever look at screens.

■ We look at screens all day and hardly ever walk.

This is The Great WFH (Working From Home) Problem in a nutshell. We sit at home and are trapped at our desk. Recent studies have demonstrated this, along with the effect it is having. Working from home due to COVID-19 was associated with more time sitting down, which was in turn negatively associated with health and well-being (9).

So we are moving less. But we've already established that studies show there is a clearly-defined mood uplift from movement and breathwork. They make us feel better. This is not going to end well unless we take action.

What follows may seem a bit simplistic. It is, but it's inspired by science.

To help us do plenty of low-level movement throughout the day, we need to set up our environment right. There is an NLP change model known as Logical Levels which tells us the easiest area in which to make lasting changes is our environment. It's easier to make changes at the level of environment than at the levels of behavior, capabilities, skills, values, beliefs or identity. We'll look at this model more later, but for now, how can you adapt your environment— home, surroundings and routine—so you can move more?

Think laterally. Move chairs away from your workspace so you have to stand up more. Leave your trainers by the door to encourage you to exercise. Buy a good umbrella. (This may at first sight not seem to qualify as a top energy tip, but I bought a good umbrella so I can walk in the London rain. It gets used often. I'll come back from a walk on a damp day with a boosted mood. I walk obsessively now, come rain or shine.) What else can you change?

Adapt your environment and routine to make it as easy as possible to move and breathe.

Ridiculously basic I know, but potentially meh-busting. Logical Levels suggests upgrading our environment is the quickest and easiest way to change. It can help encourage positive Pavlovian responses too—I see my trainers by the door, I think about going for a walk. You first consciously, then unconsciously start to incorporate more moderate exercise into your day.

In 20 years time, we may be shocked at how little we understood about how to look after ourselves in the early WFH days. Be ahead of the curve. Set up your home and surroundings to make movement easier.

References

1. Aerobic exercise for Alzheimer's disease: A randomized controlled pilot trial—https://www.ncbi.nlm.nih.gov/pmc/articles/PMC5302785/

2. Effectiveness of an Energy Management Training Course on Employee Well-Being: A Randomized Controlled Trial—https://journals.sagepub.com/doi/full/10.1177/0890117118776875

3. Relationship Among Physical Activity Level Mood and Anxiety States and Quality of Life in Physical Education Students—https://www.ncbi.nlm.nih.gov/pmc/articles/PMC5633699/

4. Why exercise alone won't save us—https://www.theguardian.com/news/2019/jan/03/why-exercise-alone-wont-save-us

5. Everyone could enjoy the "survival advantage" of elite athletes—https://www.bmj.com/content/345/bmj.e8338

6. Can Exercise Improve Cognitive Symptoms of Alzheimer's Disease?—https://agsjournals.onlinelibrary.wiley.com/doi/full/10.1111/jgs.15241

7. Reduced Exertion High-Intensity Interval Training is More Effective at Improving Cardiorespiratory Fitness and Cardiometabolic Health than Traditional Moderate-Intensity Continuous Training—https://www.mdpi.com/1660-4601/16/3/483/htm

8. Effect of Qigong on quality of life: a cross-sectional population-based comparison study in Taiwan—https://bmcpublichealth.biomedcentral.com/articles/10.1186/1471-2458-11-546

9. Working From Home and Job Loss Due to the COVID-19 Pandemic Are Associated With Greater Time in Sedentary Behaviors—https://www.ncbi.nlm.nih.gov/pmc/articles/PMC7674395/

Meh-busting Exercise Reminders...

1

Move while you work. Constant low-level exercise (or getting off your ass) throughout the day boosts your mood.

2

Use WFH workout tech. Change your brain and body and release endorphins with innovative health tech.

3

Try breath-related exercise. Increase circulation, get better sleep, and invigorate your day.

Chapter Three

Cold

66

Take cold showers, or swim outside in cold water. It gives you the feeling that you are alive.

99

WIM HOF

Why this theme?

Connecting with extreme cold temperatures can help us to increase the happy chemicals in our brain. So the temperature now plummets as we investigate all the different ways in which cold can help us to maintain a natural state of mind and body, overcome fear and feel energized.

Exposure to cold seems to switch on areas of the brain and the body that are associated with energy and healing. It's powerful in helping us to overcome fear and anxiety, maintain a natural state of mind and body, and generally feel pumped up. This is true, even though it often hurts like hell: when you get properly cold your meh will be long forgotten.

The science shows that just a cold shower can send an overwhelming quantity of electrical impulses from peripheral nerve endings to the brain, resulting in a mood boost (1). Research also shows that the cold is great for fighting aches and pains and can help you perform better (2) and a French study found that cold exposure led to a decrease in weight circumference, body weight and body mass index (3). Mind you, I tend to be ravenous after getting super cold, so I'm not sure about the weight loss bit.

There are obviously significant risks associated with exposure to the cold. Please take all the relevant safety advice, and always consult your doctor before changing your health routine.

What can you expect in this section?

We'll start with something you could do at home today—a short cold shower. Then we'll get more adventurous with a spot of cryotherapy. We'll take lessons from Mother Nature with cold plunges and wild swimming. And we'll use some simple NLP along the way so it won't feel so bad after all.

You can expect to feel instantly uplifted when you try these techniques, as well as noticing longer-term health benefits. Let's start by taking inspiration from a man who has climbed Mount Everest in a pair of shorts and open-toed sandals.

COLD SHOWERS: 30 SECONDS ISN'T THAT BAD

I have been lucky enough to explore every aspect of getting cold with the world-famous extreme athlete known as "The Ice Man," Wim Hof. Wim has done all sorts of clearly bonkers things in the cold—including setting a world record when he did indeed climb Everest in shorts.

Wim believes that by subjecting your body to the cold you can maintain a natural, primal state of mind and body. He says the real secret is combining cold exposure with focusing on the breath. He calls it conscious breathing, and says it creates more energy to help your body cope. By focusing on the breath, you also give your vascular system a workout, and (the bit we are most interested in) you ramp up the "feel good" chemicals in the brain.

Luckily, you don't have to climb Everest to harness the cold. Wim says the cheapest, quickest way to get started with the cold is in your shower. He gave me a few extra rules to make this more effective. He told me to:

■ Make the shower as cold as possible (difficult)

■ Get under there for 30 seconds (also difficult)

■ Focus on the breath (makes it a bit more bearable)

My experience is that this is a deeply unpleasant activity for the first 15 seconds or so. It is slightly less unpleasant for the next 15 seconds. And then it is impressively mood-boosting afterwards. Which makes those 30 seconds worth it.

If this is too tough you could try the "cold-ish option"—not a Wim-endorsed method but one that helps me. Just make the temperature piercing rather than polar. Or start with a regular shower—nice n' toasty, and then make it cold at the end. You'll quickly notice that you are able to tolerate the cold more and more.

DID YOU KNOW

Wim Hof has claimed the grand total of 26 Guinness World Records for his extraordinary feats, including swimming under ice for 66 meters, prolonged full-body contact with ice, and the longest ice bath (1 hour, 52 minutes and 42 seconds). He really loves the cold!

Wim allows scientists to study his methods for their research. In one study, subjects were injected with a substance designed to induce flu-like symptoms (which obviously sounds fairly unpleasant). Those participants who'd been trained in Wim's techniques—meditation, breathing techniques and immersions in ice cold water—showed fewer symptoms and an ability to control the nervous system's response more effectively (4). That means cold showers combined with breathing can help you feel less stressed and more alert, and boost your immune system.

In the interest of looking after my fellow wusses who feel the cold,

I think I should give these various methods of cold exposure a brrr rating. I give cold showers a brrr rating of 3 out of 5. Thirty seconds really isn't that bad when you feel so juicy afterwards.

CRYOTHERAPY: LIKE A QUADRUPLE ESPRESSO

Perhaps you're looking for something a bit more intense than the simple cold shower. Cryotherapy is a technique where you expose your body to extreme cold temperatures for a very short period of time. You climb into a tank and the dial gets set to minus 240 degrees Fahrenheit. It's so cold that if you stay in longer than three minutes, you risk getting frostbite.

It all clearly sounds like madness. So why on earth would you do this? That is exactly the question I was asking myself one October morning in West Hollywood, while I was waiting to get picked up by the most extreme biohacker I had met. Fashion stylist and "lifestylist" Luke Storey doesn't do things by halves, He'd planned a full day of hacking our bodies and minds. I was nervous. I had a suspicion that at least one of the activities he had planned I might not enjoy. Possibly all of them.

As we drove towards the hills, he ran me through the plan. Float tanks, four different types of sauna, an ice house, and a Kundalini yoga class. We were also going to drive for two hours out of Hollywood up to 8,000 feet above sea level to collect spring water via an elaborate system of pipes and bottles. Yes, rather than buying a bottle of spring water in the shop, Luke goes and collects it himself. The man is dedicated.

Most worryingly, I was reluctantly going to try the biohacker's favorite technique of cryotherapy for the first time. I didn't really want to do it. Why should I freeze my nuts off on a beautiful autumn day in California? I have a lanky, skinny frame. I lack insulation. My fingers and toes are like ice blocks in winter. I like heat, not cold. I'm one of the world's biggest wusses when it comes to feeling chilly. I was apprehensive that I might not be able to manage being in a chamber for three minutes while the temperature plunged to minus 240 Fahrenheit. I unsuccessfully tried to hide my skepticism, but Luke wasn't impressed. As we pulled into the cryotherapy center, he tersely responded, "You live in London, so you have no reason to be a baby about the cold."

The attendants ran me through the safety protocol as I listened in a daze. "If you have a piercing in a sensitive area below the neck, you'd best take that out or cover it up. Otherwise things might freeze off in a very painful area." *Okay!*

Why exactly was it that Luke had brought me to the intriguingly named Grotto De Sal again? He told me he loved cryotherapy, as it was effective for fighting inflammation and overcoming fears, and there was a natural mood-enhancement from the cold as well.

The door to the tank opened and a rush of mist escaped. I took off my dressing gown. This was the moment. As I clambered in, Luke chuckled. I whimpered.

The timer started. My head poked over the top of the tank so I could talk to Luke. After 15 seconds I told him I was convinced I wasn't going to make it to one minute, let alone three. Imagine going for a walk on a freezing winter's day with just underwear on. During a blizzard. That was the sensation on my skin.

Now the glacial mist was gently floating out of the tank around my face. But as the clock ticked, I started to think slightly more positive things. I'd made it to one minute thirty. Physically it hurt, but mentally I was starting to feel oddly proud that I'd lasted as long as I had. Maybe I could do this after all? There was nothing pleasurable about the physical sensation. But I started to feel something close to pride that I was a bit more resilient than I had thought.

By two minutes thirty, I knew I was going to make it. And then I really started to feel the burn. Ever lost a glove in the snow? That feeling. I closed my eyes, let out a primal roar, and resolved to stay in.

On the stroke of three minutes, the door opened. I emerged into what felt like blissful heat. The pleasant tingling warmth of the room on my skin felt delightful. And my mood? A bit like bungee-jumping and downing a quadruple espresso at the same time. I felt a sense of accomplishment having overcome my fears, as well as the huge invigorating mood-enhancement from the cold.

There aren't many things in this book that give me extra zip as instantly as cryotherapy. I give it a brrr rating of 4 out of 5. Weirdly three minutes is quite manageable, even at minus 240 Fahrenheit.

COLD TANK: THE BRRR RATING GOES UP A NOTCH

If you're looking for an extreme exposure to cold that even cryotherapy can't match, then look no further. The cold tank (aka an ice bath) will reboot your energy... if you're brave enough.

My experience with the cold tank was at a 24-hour Los Angeles institution, the Wi Korean Spa. And it came roughly five hours after the cryotherapy session. I know.

This place provides a variety of therapies to wired Hollywood residents. They alternate between the cold, and the very hot—clay saunas, jade saunas, and salt saunas releasing microscopic amounts of salt into the atmosphere (don't ask me why that is important). It's open 24/7 and apparently there's no shortage of frazzled locals looking to let off some steam in the middle of the night.

First, to the cold tank. We're not talking about a mild chill here. We're talking about Arctic cold. The most frigid ice bath you can imagine. Think: pure pain. I looked for bits of ice floating in the water. How could this be so much tougher than the cryotherapy tank?

I tried to remind myself of the reasons for getting into an ice bath: boost mood, improve recovery, and reduce inflammation (5).

The venue itself resembled a civilized Roman baths with less steam. Friends lounged in the icy waters chatting. It all seemed quite doable. I gently lowered myself into the water. And the pain began. My mind screamed. My skin crawled. I jumped out. Three seconds. Great job. It was so cold, my skin felt like it was burning. Having yelped like a chihuahua, I leapt out and declared my biohacking day over.

But it wasn't. Luke gently encouraged me back in and this time I was more resilient. One minute turned into two. And two into more. Somehow, I ended up lounging and chatting like the others in the icy burn for six minutes. Afterward I felt awesome. Again, I'd achieved something I didn't think was possible.

My reward was to step straight out of the cold plunge into the "clay sauna" with clay especially imported from Korea. This isn't particularly typical for a cold bath venue, but it was a real treat. As we immersed ourselves under the thousands of tiny clay balls on the floor of the sauna the temperature hit 220F. My mood levels had gone through the roof. Those electrical impulses from the peripheral nerve endings to my brain had been well and truly switched on.

Meh? What meh?

Try it at home for free in your bathtub. Fill with cold water and a bag of ice, and bingo, you have a cold tank.

I give cold tanks/ice baths a brrr rating of 5 out of 5. You'll still get that quadruple espresso feeling. But I have to level with you: it's tough. It's not a pleasant experience in the moment. Which is why it's all the more lovely if you can cover yourself in small hot clay balls afterwards.

WILD SWIMMING: BLUE MIND THEORY

Swimming outside in cold water is particularly good for us. Research suggests a positive link between wild swimming and mood (6), and health (7, 8). And that's before we've even get started on the relatively new, but trendy phenomenon known as Blue Mind Theory. This is a concept formulated in 2013 by marine biologist Dr Wallace J Nichols. His bestselling book Blue Mind looked at the immense impact that being near water has on our minds, bodies and emotions (9). So what is blue mind theory? He describes it as "the mildly meditative state we fall into when near, in, on or under water." It's the opposite of "red mind", which is anxious, over-connected and over-stimulated.

To put it another way; blue mind = calm and energized, red mind = meh.

In search of more "blue mind" one Saturday morning, I eagerly packed some trunks and persuaded my toddler son to get in the car for a day out. To be fair, he was 18 months old so he didn't really have much choice. I strapped him in the back seat and off we went to our local pond.

This is one of those ideas that is a lot better in theory than in practice. I don't have much of a history of wild swimming and my aim with a toddler in tow was to stay safe with more of a paddle than a full-on swim. But the start of the day was not auspicious. In fact the dip was almost immediately cancelled by the large signs around the pond, warning of toxic blue-green algae.

My son looked at me with what seemed like disdain. We were forced to get back in the car and drive to another lake close to London, charmingly called Frensham Little Pond. No signs. Phew. As we gingerly waded in, he started to get increasingly fractious. I was gently encouraged by a fully-submerged grandmother and her 14-year-old grandson. She told me they went there every day and found it to be a lovely bonding activity. I smiled politely and thought, *there's no chance you'll find me here in January.*

The honest truth is that it was mid-summer and the water was cool, but not cold. Once we were in, we seemed to ease into a more joyful mood. We started to splash and mess about in the shallows, always being mindful of safety. The water was bracing even in July but not unbearable. I felt a real connection with my son, who was admittedly clinging on tight but smiling and laughing at the same time.

Dr Nicholls says, "Water is medicine." And on that cool day in July, I felt it. I became a wild swimming convert. My meh dissolved into the lake.

Wild swimming gets a brrr rating of 5 out of 5. When it's not midsummer, it can feel colder than a cold tank. But just think how energized you will feel when you get all warm and toasty afterwards. Splashing about outside has a lot going for it.

COPE WITH COLD: PAVLOV'S DOGS CAN HELP

If you are worried, nervous or anxious about subjecting yourself to the extreme cold methods in this book, here's something that will help you cope. It is an exercise called anchoring, which will also help you generally feel less meh in cold temperatures.

But before we get onto the exercise, let's examine a sacred spiritual practice performed by Tibetan Buddhist Monks. They enter a state of deep meditation while sitting outside in freezing temperatures with very little on. To test their meditative powers, they are wrapped in a load of soaking wet sheets. Imagine sitting outside on a winter's day, wrapped in damp, cold rags. Not much fun. Incredibly, the monks not only withstand it, but end up making the sheets steam as they get warm and eventually completely dry out.

The monks use a specific breath-and-meditation routine that powerfully heats up the body from within. Whilst the breath heats up the body, they also employ a powerful visualization of flames at locations around the body accompanied by intense sensations of bodily heat in the spine.

Studies have verified the way that the monks control their inner energy to heat the sheets dry (10). For mere mortals, this could result in looking very silly at best, or serious injury if it went wrong. So, don't try this at home.

Admittedly the Tibetan Monks make the average cold exposure look a bit lightweight, but the principle is the same. Your mind and your body work together to provide a jolt of energy. The monks are using powerful breathwork to activate a more physical meditative state. The Meh Directory has some of my favorite breathing apps, books and workouts.

Here, we're going to take inspiration from the visualization the monks use alongside the breathwork. When they are thinking of the flames, they visualize heat and remember what heat feels like. This makes use of the process known in NLP as anchoring. It involves getting the brain to summon a thought or an emotion. By using anchors you can quickly start to think positive (or warm) thoughts.

The famous Russian scientist Ivan Pavlov was the first to discover this. He would ring a bell as his dogs were being fed. After a while, he could ring the bell, and his dogs would salivate even when there was no food. A stimulus (in this case food, then the bell summoning the thought of food) could illicit an automatic response.

I love the concept of anchoring and I notice it everywhere. Here are some examples of anchors that elicit strong feelings in me.

▓ A favorite song that reminds me of a gig

▓ The smell of coffee

▓ Pictures of a relaxing time with my family

And now, we can take inspiration from Pavlov to cope with cold exposure more effectively.

Anchoring technique to help you deal with the cold

▓ Think of a time when you felt warm and relaxed. Maybe you were on holiday. Make it a good memory.

▓ Fully associate with this memory. Remember exactly what you could see. Make the colors bright and vivid. How did it sound where you were? Turn the volume up? And how did that heat feel on your skin? Really enjoy that feeling?

■ As you do this, touch your two index fingers together.

■ Whenever you want to feel warmer in future, touch your two index fingers together again. You are now using the technique of anchoring to start feeling warm.

Here's my favorite way of using this method. At night in winter, when I get into bed my toes are sometimes cold, I'll use anchoring, and within a couple of minutes I will start to feel the heat flooding in. It's a magical process to be able to heat the body up with nothing but thought.

Remember: when you are about to get seriously cold, touch your index fingers together. Allow yourself to focus on the memory once again. Anchoring means you will automatically start to feel those same sensations that you felt when you were warm.

Let's end this section with a Wim Hof quote. He says, "Unless you are willing to experience new things, you will never realize your full potential." So give as many of these suggestions as you can a go, just once, and see how you feel. You'll never know otherwise.

References

1. Adapted cold shower as a potential treatment for depression— https://pubmed.ncbi.nlm.nih.gov/17993252/

2. Whole-Body Cryotherapy: Potential to Enhance Athlete Preparation for Competition?—https://www.ncbi.nlm.nih.gov/pmc/articles/PMC6691163/

3. Mechanism Underlying Tissue Cryotherapy to Combat Obesity/ Overweight: Triggering Thermogenesis—https://www.ncbi.nlm.nih.gov/pmc/articles/PMC5954866/

4. Voluntary activation of the sympathetic nervous system and attenuation of the innate immune response in humans—https://www.wimhofmethod.com/uploads/kcfinder/files/PNAS.pdf

5. An add-on training program involving breathing exercises, cold exposure, and meditation attenuates inflammation and disease activity in axial spondyloarthritis—A proof of concept trial—https://journals.plos.org/plosone/article?id=10.1371/journal.pone.0225749

6. Open water swimming as a treatment for major depressive disorder—https://casereports.bmj.com/content/2018/bcr-2018-225007

7. Swimming in Ireland: Immersions in therapeutic blue space—https://www.sciencedirect.com/science/article/abs/pii/S1353829214001452?via=ihub

8. Swimming as an accretive practice in healthy blue space— https://www.sciencedirect.com/science/article/abs/pii/S1755458615300591?via=ihub

9. Blue Mind Research & References Collected reports and publications related to and cited in Blue Mind—https://www.wallacejnichols.org/467/bluemind-research.html

10. Drying Wet Towels On Naked Bodies At -25C—https://www.advaita-academy.org/blogs/drying-wet-towels-on-naked-bodies-at-25-deg-c-g-tummo-meditation/

Meh-busting Cold Reminders...

1

**Take a 30-second cold shower.
Good for increasing the "feel good"
'chemicals in the brain.**

2

**Try Cryotherapy. The quadruple
espresso option. Overcome fear and
feel a sense of accomplishment.**

3

**Go Wild Swimming.
Maintain a natural state of mind
and body and improve your mood.**

Chapter Four

Mind

"

Fuck nudes, send me a dated invoice from your therapist so I know you're working on yourself.

@WITTYIDIOT ON INSTAGRAM

"

Why this theme?

It's time to switch on our brain, access deeper states and unleash our potential.

Sometimes the same old meh appears in our lives and we can't shake it off. It can be low energy or brain fog. Or it can go deeper—something locked inside our mind that holds us back. The same old problems crop up time and again, leaving us feeling down and depressed. We don't resolve our more deeply held fears and anxieties which keep producing the same results.

Let's make a commitment to delving into the mind and changing that meh for good. It'll give us a long-term boost.

What can you expect in this section?

Here's what we'll do in this part of the book:

▧ Switch on our brain.

▧ Reclaim our natural sharpness and vitality.

▧ Go deep, using cutting-edge innovation.

▧ Make lasting changes.

The main theme of this section is something I call a mind pyramid. The relationship between your mind and the world is like a pyramid. At the bottom, you've got the stuff that is easier to change, like behavior and environment. At the top, you have the deep stuff—values, beliefs, and then identity. This section takes the mind on a ride up the pyramid.

This is based on the effective NLP technique known as Logical Levels, which I have mentioned before. It helps the mind understand how it relates to the world. I'm going to break it down and adapt it to help us optimize our mind and energy. We'll make it super easy, and I'm going to call it our "mind pyramid".

MIND PYRAMID

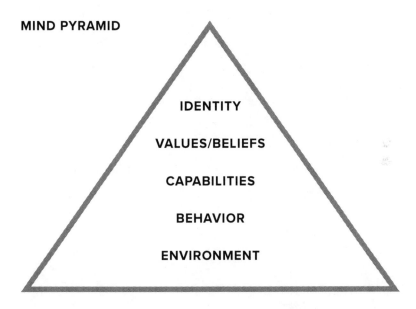

We'll start our ride with some easy wins at the bottom of the pyramid. We'll adapt our environment and behavior to help our mind. We'll get some immediate wins in energy and mood. Then we'll climb up to the more challenging areas. We'll do some work on ourselves as we activate our brain and harness our brainwaves, use neurofeedback, access deeper states, and unleash our potential. When we get to the very top of the pyramid, we'll address fundamental questions about our deeper identity. That will help us to discover our true inner vitality and identity.

We'll want to address throughout the section why that same old meh keeps appearing, and make sure it stays away.

DECLUTTER YOUR MIND: SIMPLICITY IS THE ULTIMATE SOPHISTICATION

Life is way too complicated these days. There are a million and one things that need to be done at once, and our poor little minds can't cope.

If only we knew how to simplify and declutter our minds. Luckily, in a cave somewhere, they found the Ten Commandments of Clutter.

These tongue-in-cheek rules are at the bottom of the mind pyramid, so potentially the easiest to change quickly. So, let's declutter our environment and our minds.

1. Thou shalt take at least 5-10 minutes a day to just chill and do nothing.

2. Thou shalt focus on one thing at once. If necessary, switch thy iPhone off to do this.

3. Thou shalt simplify your schedule. Cut non-essential clutter to free up time, energy and brainpower.

4. Thou shalt throw stuff away. (Physical clutter = mind clutter.)

5. Thou shalt only have three windows open on your computer at any one time. (Too many windows open will always do thy head in.)

6. Thou shalt get enough sleep. (Lack of sleep is often related to a fuzzy mind.)

7. Thou shalt be aware that when thou browses ye olde Facebook and Twitter, your mind becomes engaged in "continuous partial attention", otherwise known as not focusing properly on anything.

8. Thou shalt remember that the best things in life don't have a screen.

9. Thou shalt take time to just think: "When you are doing the least work, you are the most active."

10. Thou shalt remember the words of Leonardo Da Vinci: "Simplicity is the ultimate sophistication."

ESCAPE THE SCREENS: 20% LESS MEH

Many of us now spend more time everyday gazing into screens than we do into the eyes of real life, wonderful, unpredictable human beings.

Perhaps it's time to escape the screens and escape the meh.

We are still at the bottom of our mind pyramid here, in the area known as "environment". Altering our surroundings is one of the easiest ways to make positive psychological changes.

Many of the suggestions in this book involve making use of the glories of modern technology. We can access it to get our brains into a more primal, relaxed state, and activate the parasympathetic nervous system—the part of your physiology that helps you decrease anxiety.

But I also encourage you to remove the tech from around you at select times. I kept an exciting spreadsheet for years detailing my energy levels. And one big secret emerged as being far more effective than anything else:

Switching off screens increased my energy levels by up to 20%.

Clearly this was not a randomized controlled study, but the results are still significant. The more I escaped technology during the day, the more lively I felt. When I escaped devices for a big chunk of time—more than eight hours or so—I was way more energized or, to put it another way, I felt around 20% less meh. I'm convinced most people will get the same benefits. Slightly more formal research than my own metrics is still developing in this area, but a link has been found between screentime and a slightly increased risk of anxiety and depression (1).

Some people like to do this by switching off for an hour or two each day. That's what I do. I'm out of contact for a portion of the day. It's annoying for people who are trying to reach me, but great for my poor overworked brain which gets a breather. I use the Airplane mode or Downtime mode on my devices to help. Unfortunately many people have to be connected throughout the working week, but some still choose a "Screen-free Saturday" or a "Screen-free Sunday", which they often report to be the best day of their week.

We recharge when we're actually living, looking at real people, engaging in life and not being illuminated by the glow of our phones. Then you are in the perfect position to make use of the power of technology at select moments. The thought of a whole day without screens sounds like bliss. So why don't we do it more often? Trust me, your day becomes more yay.

READ SMARTER: COMPOUND INTEREST ON YOUR LEARNINGS

Books enrich our lives. In the days and weeks after reading something inspiring (like, perhaps even this book?) we are motivated to take action and implement these lessons into our lives. However, we often find that feeling doesn't last. We forget what we've learnt.

How can we keep this inspiration fresh, way into the future?

The first problem we need to combat is this: we forget what we've read and learned. The psychological phenomenon of recency bias is a cognitive bias that means we favor recent events over historic ones. When it comes to books, it means we forget books we read a long time ago, even if they had a powerful message. Will you remember all the tips from this book in a year's time? Will you remember any? Recency bias means that, in the future, the message of this book and other good ones you've read will not be so fresh in your mind.

But not any more. We're about to give you an upgrade.at the behavior level of the mind pyramid.

There is a way to beat this memory bias. You use tech to keep the books you love top-of-mind, and to keep that "just read" vibe—even when you finished a book years ago. You do this by learning from your highlights.

Step 1: Make highlights on anything you read online, including Kindle books.

Step 2: Get daily highlights of your own personalized best bits.

I get daily personalized quotes from Readwise. It's an effective way to continue to learn from the books you've read. It's a simple idea. It syncs up with your Kindle highlights, then sends you a daily email. You choose how many quotes you get a day. Impressively, it will also work with print books by cleverly transcribing text from photos. There are alternatives such as Klib, Clippings and Booky.

Today, I received a quote from Yuval Noah Harari's book, Homo Deus. I read it over a year ago on Kindle, and of course, had totally forgotten the passage I'd highlighted. Don't have a Kindle? Prefer to read actual books? No problem. You can scan print pages and it will convert the text. Then you read the quotes on app or desktop.

When you read an energizing or inspiring part of a book, you'll get the benefit of it way into the future. This is tech at its best—enhancing your mind with books over and over again.

FLOAT TANKS: FLOAT INTO THE FUTURE

Float tanks offer an hour of sensory deprivation to restore mind and body. In the pitch-black silence, you'll float effortlessly for an hour with no sense of sight, sound, or touch, as the water is the same temperature as the air. We're still at the behavior level of the mind pyramid, but when you ease away the concerns of the day this way, you might go deeper than you ever have before.

The research on floating is seriously impressive. It shows that floating improves people's energy levels and overall happiness, and makes us feel more "optimistic". It also induces a deep state of relaxation and helps us sleep (2).

This definitely is one of the "bit of a hassle" options in the search for more energy. By the time you've traveled to the float center, paid your money, got undressed, put earplugs in, and settled into a large pod with half a ton of Epsom salts to help you bob on the surface, you have invested a lot of time and effort into your relaxation session for the day.

As an occasional treat, it's fun and a nice addition to your routine. And perhaps it'll be more. I have friends who have transcended to entirely different levels of consciousness in the tank. It's one of their favorite activities in the world.

As you know, in this book I like to offer cheap alternatives all the way through. Unfortunately this is not something you can replicate in your bath at home—you'll drown if you do!

Remember to collect metrics when you float, to see if it's something you want to incorporate into your long-term vitality regime. If you don't want to spend as much as it costs to float, the following technique is an easier way to get a similar boost. It won't cost you a penny. And you'll be a lot drier afterwards.

BINAURAL BEATS: HARNESS YOUR BRAINWAVES FOR LESS THAN THE PRICE OF A CUP OF COFFEE

Scientists have learned to not only measure what's going on in the brain, but to change it too.

There are five most commonly analyzed types of human brainwaves: Delta (0.5 to 4Hz); Theta (4 to 7Hz); Alpha (8 to 12Hz); Beta (13 to 30Hz); and Gamma (30 to 80Hz) (3). They all move at different speeds. These fluctuate within our brain throughout the day, depending on what we are doing. And it turns out we can give them a little nudge.

The simplest way to do this, and a fun place to start, is by experimenting with binaural beats. This alone can help you to start busting "meh" brainwave states during the day, and to feel more restful at night (4). Binaural beats tracks or apps, which play odd sounds at different frequencies, are proven to induce altered states of consciousness such as more of an Alpha state (reducing stress and anxiety—a proper chill-out zone), or a Gamma state (the ideas zone—for memory processing, language, learning).

Your brain will literally start to work at a different speed as a result.

Many of these apps also revel in titling their various programs in gloriously trippy ways. It makes it all the more fun. I use an app simply called Binaural Beats. The sound is quite distracting. However, you can play other stuff like music at the same time which masks it a little while it still does its work. You would think this sounds like two kinds of loud noises drowning each other out, but it kind of works.

You will want to play around with the different settings. For instance, while I was writing this section I had Alpha/Relaxation/Dreams setting at 8 Hz playing dance music in the background. Despite the uplifting music, the Alpha brainwaves were way too relaxing. That would be lovely before bed, but I started to drift off as I was writing. So, then I cranked up the dial to some Beta brainwaves at 16.5Hz (the wide awake zone—in which you are focused and "on it") and I now feel considerably more alert. Some say the brain gets used to the tones after a while and the effect then becomes less powerful. So see how it works for you.

You can use binaural beats to both revitalize and recharge. You can turn your energy up or down depending on the time of day. In the morning, travel through your brainwave frequencies to a renewed sense of vitality. And then when you want to recharge, travel back down to something more peaceful.

MEDITATION: WORKING ON OUR GOLDFISH BRAIN

Meditation has come a long way over the last few years: increasingly mainstream and less woo-woo. It's becoming more and more acceptable to tell the world you meditate. And why not?

Meditation can change the structure and function of the brain. That means we've moved up the mind pyramid to capabilities. When using meditation, you are looking at a whole laundry list of benefits (5), including;

■ Increase in focus

■ Improvements in learning and concentration

■ Better memory and attention span

■ Stronger immune system

■ Greater physical and psychological resilience

■ Reduction in stress, anxiety, and depression

■ Better sleep

Meditation expert Dan Harris cautioned me that meditation is not a magic pill. It isn't suddenly going to make everything better. But it does make you, in his words, "10% happier". And the busier you are, the more you'll appreciate this sweet downtime.

Taking ten minutes out for some kind of meditation during the day is like a circuit breaker for my mind, or a drink of water for the brain. I find it a very important chance to reset my energy levels, and crucially, to reset my focus.

There are many different ways you can do this. You can sit quietly and focus on your breathing for ten minutes. You can also use affordable audio programs, or apps that will guide you through it. The ones that I use are Sam Harris's Waking Up, and Dan Harris's 10% Happier. (Maybe I need to bring out my own app called 20% Less Meh.)

These apps will make a big difference to your day, and may get you thinking about all sorts of trippy consciousness concepts. Each session tends to be about ten minutes which is manageable even in a busy schedule.

As well as apps, there is a growing market in technology designed to help you to meditate. There are headbands that take you into different brainwave states, necklaces that vibrate, and apps that play sound frequencies at different pitches into each ear. It's all designed to deepen your meditative state. You could even try the Sensate meditation pebble to see if it works for you. You hang it round your neck and it sends weird vibrations through your chest up into your head. It uses "the science of bone conduction" to send these vibrations up into your body, a bit like a gentle bass speaker. Yes, it sounds odd, but it's very relaxing, and I have found it to be a nice addition to my meditation routine when I want to prioritize deep relaxation.

There are lots of technological (and non-technological) solutions for meditation. Test them all out and collect metrics, remembering the importance of the NLP maxim: Do What Works.

When you meditate regularly, the science suggests you'll have more energy and become less stressed.

EFT: TAPPING ON FACE AND BODY

Many of us live in a permanent state of over-stimulation. We're "a bit too hyper". We find it hard to relax, even when we know it is so important. Author Sharon Salzberg says "I don't believe we can survive for long in a state of constant agitation. Our bodies and hearts need rest to replenish stores of energy."

Emotional Freedom Therapy (EFT, also known as "Tapping") can replenish those stores of energy.

It draws its power from the ancient wisdom of traditional Chinese medicine. And decidedly modern scientific studies back up its power. Clinical EFT improves multiple physiological markers of health and well-being and leads to a reduction in stress too (6). Personally, it helps me get less hyper. That's not a particularly technical way of describing what's going on, but it's true.

It's one of the quickest ways you can switch off the agitation and start to replenish that energy at a behavioral level. It's known as "energy psychology", and can help with deep change, so it also now helps us climb the pyramid to explore our values and beliefs.

It's no exaggeration to say that, when I spent three months ill in bed, this was the discovery that helped me start to get on the road back to health. After my illness in the jungle, I used tapping for years with genuinely incredible results. I still do. It helped me to learn a lot about myself. It is so powerful for me, it feels quite private to even write about it. But—who cares—I just want you to know about the potential of tapping as well.

It involves somebody tapping on your face and body. Don't let that put you off. You can do it yourself if you'd prefer. The fingers tap on energy meridians that are situated just beneath the surface of the skin. By focusing on the body, you start to tune into the intrinsic link between body and mind. Doing so can unlock the emotions stored in the body. You can make a start now:

■ Step One: Focus on an issue that is concerning you. For instance, it might be a relationship issue, a health issue, or a work issue. Keep thinking about that issue as you take two fingers and tap a few times on the karate chop point of your hand. Then tap;

1. Above your eye

2. On the side of your eye

3. Below your eye

4. Between your nose and mouth

5. Below your mouth

6. On your chest (close to collarbone)

7. Under your arm, below armpit

8. On the top of your head

■ Step Two: Repeat 1-8 a few times, still thinking about the issue. How do you feel about the issue now?

That's Tapping 101. There is plenty more to it, of course, but you've made a start already. I love it so much, I did some training in it. I learnt more about its immense power, and how it can help us to work our way up the mind pyramid to do some deeper work on ourselves.

You'll make quicker progress if you work with a skilled practitioner, as I have for many years. That work can also provide some deep revelations at the level of values and beliefs and even identity, as well as simple energy shifts.

I like to tap when I've finished an intense day on-air in the studio. I'll leave work, ease into the car, and start tapping. It gently takes my mind to a less frenetic place. And I'll also tap in quieter, more reflective moments for deep inner work and revelations.

OTHER WAYS TO TAP

There are a number of ways to tap into the ancient wisdom of energy meridians. Here's a fun one. My friend, Chinese medicine practitioner and bestselling author Katie Brindle, gave me a bamboo "tapper". It's very strange. It looks a little bit like she found it in a dungeon somewhere. She told me it's the way the Chinese have super-charged their energy levels for years. Search for bamboo tappers. Then tap all over the body in a daily ritual. Go briskly and firmly. It'll invigorate your senses, brain and body.

NEUROFEEDBACK: MORE CALM. SHARPER FOCUS. BETTER SLEEP.

Neurofeedback works by measuring your brainwaves (the same delta, theta, alpha, beta and gamma we looked at in the binaural beats section). Those brainwaves are then encouraged to behave differently. Think of it as a bit like a gym workout for the brain.

Research shows you can use neurofeedback to boost your attention, spatial rotation, complex psychomotor skills, implicit procedural memory, recognition memory, perceptual binding, intelligence, mood and well-being (7). In other words, it'll make you feel less meh right now. But it'll also help us climb right to the top of the pyramid, as you'll see in a moment.

First though, let's experiment with neurofeedback. To do this properly, you'll need to use an EEG (electroencephalogram).

Here's where tech is our friend.

A few years ago, you needed a second mortgage to own anything that could perform the role of an EEG. Happily, there are now more affordable ways to try neurofeedback. There are now various "wearable EEGs" on the market, which start at $200 (approx £150).

These devices aim to take you on a trippy journey to a different place. They also "gamify" meditation which might well work for you if you are a competitive so-and-so like me. I sometimes use a Muse "brain-sensing headband" that uses EEG. This provides a surprising level of in-depth mental discovery. This device admittedly makes you look quite strange, so don't plan a trip to the shops while wearing it. You start by putting your headband on, then select a program on the app and allow your mind to gently drift off to a different place. As the program continues, you hear a series of different sounds depending on how "well" you are doing. Afterwards, you check your scores.

It's so accessible and accurate it's been used by numerous research projects at prestigious institutions including Harvard. It's a great option for re-energizing. But there is neurofeedback technology that is even more powerful than that.

One of the strangest experiences I've had over the past few years had me clutching my backpack outside a mysterious mountain retreat near Seattle called "40 Years of Zen". I had arrived for a week of electrical brain stimulation.

This was not going to be your average holiday.

I was there for the deepest possible dive into neurofeedback. I was there to climb to the top of the mind pyramid. I'd been encouraged to go there by the inventor of Bulletproof Coffee and the "father of biohacking" Dave Asprey.

He'd made a big claim. He'd told me that after a week of the hyper-advanced neurofeedback machines here, my mind would be able to access deep states of calm similar to someone who's been meditating for 40 years. Who needs to join a monastery for a lifetime when you can do the whole lot in seven days? Talk about delving into my very identity.

The daily routine was this: I would enter the pod, and then be forced to sit still as I had cold goo (conductive gel) smeared all over my scalp. Had I really paid the price of a new kitchen for a greasy scalp? Then a number of electrodes were firmly attached to my skull with wires heading to a nearby computer. Large headphones were placed over my ears and the lights switched off. Over the course of the week, I worked on improving my alpha brainwaves, which help to cultivate a calm, relaxed state. And more importantly, I did some serious deep work on myself. In the pods, we used a special technique to go through all the most difficult and traumatic moments in our pasts.

After a particularly tough pod session, Dave and I sat down with a buttery Bulletproof Coffee (coffee, MCT oil, and butter—good for energy). He told me he comes here once a month. Mind you, it is his company, and the eye-wateringly high price meant I was definitely there for a one-off. He believes it's completely changed his life, and is worth every penny. As he said, "Would you want to drive a car with an engine that ran only half as well as it was designed to?"

After having had my brain mapped for a week, I did feel like I had tapped into something deep. I'd started to examine my values, beliefs and identity and reaffirm what was important to me. I genuinely felt like I understood myself more. Something was working better and more clearly. That translated into a prolonged vitality boost after my trip.

EEGs were originally used in the fields of psychology, medicine and neuroscience. Now they're fast becoming available to ordinary people through technology like Muse. Unfortunately, I can't provide a free neurofeedback option. Regardless, it is well worth looking into for insights at the top of our mind pyramid.

DEEP WORK: WHERE'S THAT DATED INVOICE FROM YOUR THERAPIST?

'Working on yourself' takes lots of different forms. It thankfully does not mean you have to get a dated invoice from your therapist (though I love the quote), or book a week at *40 Years Of Zen*. It does, however, mean committing to making a start on climbing to the top the pyramid and understanding the deeper recesses of your brain. It is truly important to explore who you are and what your purpose is in life. It is well-documented that working with a psychologist, psychotherapist or other expert produces positive long-term outcomes (8). That means personal exploration might be the most effective long-term approach to banishing your meh forever.

This is certainly my experience. Without taking you through a blow-by-blow account of my years speaking to a psychotherapist (you'll be pleased to hear), I can tell you it has freed up my mind. It's allowed me to understand myself more and have better relationships. I'm less anxious, and more present.

Deep work doesn't have to be done with a therapist. It could be a retreat, a support group, even a book. Anything which allows you to explore your brain and your background, and how they knit together.

I believe this "deep work" is particularly important because of the challenging times we live in. Our mind and our energy are inextricably linked, while our brains are pulled in more directions than ever before. We're so frazzled in the moment we don't have time to do the deep work. So, it's worth taking some personal responsibility in this area. We have to own it. You've already started to do that by reading this book. But, what's next? How can you take more responsibility for what's going on in your head?

We understand so little about the link between the mind and our energy. But we know it's there. Gaining insights into the weird, unpredictable ways our mind works is the key to making it work better.

As we finish this section on the mind, consider this quote from motivational speaker Brendon Burchard, "Slow down. Be intentional. Notice the energy you are bringing into this space and moment. In times of chaos, commit to THIS: I'm going to role model the energy I wish the world had. You might not be able to change what is happening around you— but you can always change your reaction. Your energy is your choice."

References

1. Is screen time associated with anxiety or depression in young people? Results from a UK birth cohort—https://www.ncbi.nlm.nih.gov/pmc/articles/PMC6337855/

2. Flotation restricted environmental stimulation therapy (REST) as a stress-management tool: A meta-analysis—https://www.tandfonline.com/doi/abs/10.1080/08870440412331337093

3. EEG Normal Waveforms—https://www.ncbi.nlm.nih.gov/books/NBK539805/

4. Auditory Beat Stimulation and its Effects on Cognition and Mood States—https://www.ncbi.nlm.nih.gov/pmc/articles/PMC4428073/

5. How Meditation Can Help You Focus—https://sps.columbia.edu/news/how-meditation-can-help-you-focushttps://bmcpublichealth.biomedcentral.com/articles/10.1186/1471-2458-13-119

6. Clinical EFT (Emotional Freedom Techniques) Improves Multiple Physiological Markers of Health https://www.ncbi.nlm.nih.gov/pmc/articles/PMC6381429/

7. EEG-neurofeedback for optimising performance. I: A review of cognitive and affective outcome in healthy participants—https://www.sciencedirect.com/science/article/abs/pii/S0149763413002248?via=ihub

8. Positive psychology interventions: a meta-analysis of randomized controlled studies—https://bmcpublichealth.biomedcentral.com/articles/10.1186/1471-2458-13-119

Meh-busting Mind Reminders...

1

Simplify. Cut the physical and mental clutter. Switch on your brain. No more "continuous partial attention".

2

**Harness your brainwaves.
Use binaural beats to feel sharp.
Choose more focus, energy, or calm.**

3

**Try neurofeedback.
Access deeper states.
Unleash your deep potential.
Make deep changes.**

Chapter Five

Fuel

> **High-performing people know that getting their food right is the number one human upgrade.**

DAVE ASPREY

Why this theme?

When you get your refueling right, you'll feel invigorated and energized. But put the wrong fuel in the tank, and your energy levels will sputter to a halt. So in this section we follow some fuel timings, fuel rules, and specific fuel boosters (supplements) for mood, memory, immunity and energy.

With food, there are some things we can agree on. Vegetables, for example, tend to be less inflammatory than deep-fried doughnuts. But after that, there are differences in the way we eat our food that can have a massive impact. Some small changes around eating habits make a massive meh difference.

That's where I come in. As a journalist and biohacker, I've enjoyed grappling with the shifting science over the past six years. I've sought out the world's top experts to try and gain some objectivity on the best diet for revitalizing and re-energizing yourself. It's my job to seek out the best information and cut through the considerable noise around diet and health.

What can you expect in this section?

I've found there are three key areas we can look at to boost our vitality levels.

1. Fuel timings

2. Fuel rules

3. Fuel boosters

We'll look at the radical new research on when you eat, what you eat, and how you *supplement it.* This will all help minimize those sneaky snaccidents and give you extra oomph at the same time. Always work responsibly with your practitioner before changing your diet. It's important to me that we aim for grounded, balanced, mindful long-term change.

You won't find too much advice from me around *what* to eat because I believe many of us have very different dietary requirements. But one of the best ways we can re-energize is by looking at *when* we eat.

INTERMITTENT FASTING: BYE BYE BREAKFAST

A snaccident is inadvertently eating a whole bag of crisps when you intended to only have one or two. It's eating the full pizza when you meant to just have a slice. I'm prone to snaccidents. Most of us are. This part of the book will help you if you are a snaccidenter.

The most consistently important part of your fuel strategy may be surprising, as it doesn't focus on what you eat. Time and time again the experts have told me:

Focus more on when you eat than what you eat.

There is an ever-accumulating body of substantial scientific evidence behind intermittent fasting. This is simply eating less often. A recent study showed intermittent fasting works as effectively as diets (1). This means all those diets we struggled with over the years could just as easily have been replaced with missing a meal a day.

Intermittent fasting can help with mood (2) as well as waistline. It's also been found to:

- Improve memory

- Decrease blood pressure and resting heart rates

- Improve resistance to stress

- Modify risk factors associated with obesity

All of this science is thanks to a process known as metabolic switching, and one of the best ways you can kick start that is giving breakfast the swerve.

So did you have for breakfast today? Could you have held off on eating until lunch? Might that have given you more energy?

The purpose is to allow your digestion to recover, and your body to renew. But it also means there's simply less time in the day for snaccidents. Win-win. This isn't scientific, but personally speaking I find these little slip-ups don't seem quite so tempting outside my feeding window, in the morning at least. Those hunger pangs don't pop up in quite the same way.

I wanted help navigating the minefield of eating less often. So I approached Dr. Jason Fung. He's a world-leading expert on intermittent fasting and low-carb diets, especially when they are used for treating people with type 2 diabetes. Drawing on his scientific background, he co-wrote the bible on intermittent fasting, The Complete Guide To Fasting.

He explained to me that fasting is an ancient secret, and it's really not about starving yourself. The theory is that, by avoiding food for a bit longer every day, you increase energy (or ketones) and reduce cravings.

How to do it

■ When intermittent fasting, try thinking of your day's food intake as two meals, not three.

■ Choose breakfast and lunch, or lunch and dinner.

■ Aim for a 14-17 hour intermittent fast.

This has been my routine for many years. I tend to fast for 17 hours every day, though I know some people like to make that window shorter. I'll finish dinner by 7pm, and I won't eat breakfast. Missing breakfast is the key for me. Then I have an earlyish lunch about midday, and boom, that's my 17 hours done.

Intermittent fasting suits my personality as, on the average day, I find it tough to avoid aimlessly heading for the fridge every five minutes. And I have to be absolutely honest with you, that is still the case. But... not before my first meal of the day.

This style of eating clearly agrees with some people more than others. As I said, do work with your practitioner when changing your diet. Then collect metrics to help them assess your progress.

It's intriguing that on the health rollercoaster I've ridden for the last few years, most of the experts I've met in the health field tend to fast intermittently. That includes many of the scientists. In fact, very few still eat breakfast. Harvard Professor of Genetics Dr. David Sinclair told me he uses the practice. Add in names like Dr. Satchin Panda, Dave Asprey, Ben Greenfield and many other luminaries in this world of radical health and you realize how compelling the research is on fasting and longevity. Max Lowery invented the 2-Meal Day program, and he told me this about intermittent fasting:

"I enjoy eating large meals and feeling satisfied after eating. If I were to eat three large meals with snacks in between I would certainly be consuming more than I was burning. Two meals a day has allowed me to stay lean effortlessly, all year round."

You might feel a little under the weather while your body adjusts to fasting. Dr. Mattson observed rather drily in his paper, "Patients should be advised that feeling hungry and irritable is common initially and usually passes after two weeks to a month." But hang in there. Intermittent fasting has changed the way I refuel and has made the biggest difference to how I recharge. It boosts my energy levels every day. And I can still indulge in a good full English breakfast (a British tradition that is hard to give up). I just skip dinner instead.

FASTING TIPS

- Drink electrolytes from brands like LMNT or Seeking Health to help your body adjust to fasting.

- Use the app "Zero" for inspiration and to understand what is happening inside your body.

- Remind yourself you are getting closer to your long-term goal of more energy and focus.

LONGER FASTS: FIVE DAYS OF TORTURE?

So far we have looked at the relatively short fasts known as intermittent fasting. You might want to try something longer. Multiday fasts can provide a significant well-being and health boost (3) but can you imagine eating nothing for five days? No, me neither.

Enter The 5-Day Fasting Mimicking Diet, something created by a brilliant longevity expert called Dr. Valter Longo. It's not an actual fast, but your body thinks it is. You still get to eat stuff. Woohoo. Not much, but enough to stop your stomach loudly complaining for days on end.

Fasting mimicking perfectly mimics an actual fast, with all the benefits (4) but with enough calories to safely keep you going.

What will you get if you do this? One of the benefits of fasting is its ability to spark a process known as autophagy. This is essentially a clearing out of the old damaged cells in the body that you don't need any more. It's a bit like tidying up the house—a necessary process that keeps things nice. The longer you spend tidying the house, the more sparkling it is, and the more you'll be energized.

It's not what you'll be used to though. Typically we eat around 2000-2500 calories per day, but you only eat between 600-800 calories a day when you are fasting mimicking. The meals are light. An afternoon snack may consist of 12 almonds. And then it's a long time until your light soup dinner.

If your experience is like mine, you'll feel depleted at times during this process. It's important to note my energy was lower during parts of this fast, but supercharged afterwards. It's not an instant energy hack, but think of it as "pain today to feel awesome tomorrow".

How do you do the 5-day fasting mimicking diet? You can either cook everything yourself with exact measurements, or take the lazy option and use a company such as ProLon (linked to Dr. Longo) who'll supply everything you need for the week, all boxed up and ready-to-go. A typical day might be;

▪ Nut bar for breakfast

▪ Soup for lunch

▪ Crackers or a few olives for a snack

▪ More soup for dinner (this diet is big on soup)

▪ Nut bar for dessert

▪ Teas/special drinks/supplements throughout the day

Once you've gotten through the fasting mimicking, you will also probably be significantly trimmer. In a clinical study, ProLon was shown over three cycles to help individuals lose an average of 5.7 lbs and 1.6 inches off their waist circumference (4). This is actually one of the reasons I don't do this more regularly. There's not much weight to lose from my beanpole figure, but obviously the weight loss bit holds major appeal for many people.

You can follow Dr Longo's ProLon Diet (there's a link in the Meh Directory) for around $300 (£200) for the five days. Do it safely and always with professional guidance. It's not for the faint-hearted.

DEVELOPING HEALTHY HABITS AROUND FOOD

Another way to avoid snack slip-ups is with what I call "betterisms". This is my made-up word for something that relates to the simple NLP technique of reframing. When something doesn't go my way, I don't ask what went wrong. I ask for a betterism instead.

"What could I do better next time? How could I react differently in future?"

In this way, you reframe something that was "bad" into something that you can learn from. When it comes to food, it's possible your betterisms might include "removing the source of snacks from the house", "buying nuts instead of cookies", or "working with a practitioner to create a healthy outlook on food".

Betterisms—or turning failure into success—are important in every area of life. Roland Macy couldn't have made a success of Macy's store in New York if he hadn't learnt how to do better from his seven previous failed shops. He learnt from his mistakes, and built it better.

OPTIMIZE COFFEE: UPGRADE YOUR MORNING VITALITY

Coffee is the Superbowl of drinks. It's the cup of happiness most of us don't want to go without. It gives us an immediate boost, and improves our health. It is associated with a reduced risk of cardiovascular disease, lower incidence of diabetes, and better memory, as well as a reduced risk for Alzheimer's (5, 6, 7, 8).

But it turns out not all coffee is created equal. There can be problems with toxins, low quality beans and even micro-plastics. We'll focus here on picking the right coffee and preparing it in the right way. And you'll get even more of a morning upgrade.

When we were on holiday recently, we had a coffee capsule machine in our room. What a treat. But by the end of the week, I was convinced these capsules were giving me allergy symptoms. After every coffee, I'd quite quickly feel stuffed up and blocked. Attractive right? The problem may be that most coffee capsules are made with elements of plastic. When that plastic gets heated to high temperatures it might leach into the coffee. It certainly makes me feel like rubbish. Exactly the opposite effect I am looking for from my morning jolt of caffeine.

Plastics in food and drink are a big problem. One research paper estimated we each ingest as many as 74,000 microplastic particles each year (9) and many argue that ingesting these chemicals is harmful for our long-term health. Add in the waste aspect of coffee pods—there are 20 billion capsules currently consumed every year, apparently enough to circle the Earth 14 times, with a lot of packaging for a tiny amount of coffee.

So, here are some ideas on how to make energizing coffee choices for yourself and the planet too.

1. Drink organic coffee. Many people report feeling considerably better for it and less jittery. I do. I like Bulletproof Coffee Beans—low-toxin, low-mold, organic coffee grown by reputable farmers. Recently, I have noticed other organic and low-toxin coffees are also doing a great job. There are plenty of brands out there if you search for "low-toxin coffee". My favorite in the UK is Mindful Coffee: it has a nice buttery taste. (There are some links in the Meh Directory).

2. Yes, yes, I know you don't want to throw out your coffee capsule machine. I get that. Here's a solution: a genius somewhere invented the concept of stainless steel coffee capsules that fit perfectly into most machines. Pack your capsule with your beautiful, low-mold,

low-toxin ground coffee and stick it snugly in the machine. And it works. Then you just rinse it out and use it all over again. You will get a clean energy hit, and I've just halved the amount you spend on coffee. The environment will thank you too.

So far so good. But can we still have coffee while we fast?

This is one of the age-old questions. Many health enthusiasts anxiously ask it on a regular basis. I've obsessively tried to get this question answered. (Can you tell that I like my coffee?) Perhaps the most respected expert who has given me an answer was the world-famous Dr. Satchin Panda, author of The Circadian Code.

He told me some black coffee while fasting is fine. But... he did say his advice was based on a hunch rather than science. He said it's a grey area. In fact, he believes it'll be impossible in his lifetime to carry out a randomized controlled study to answer this question. He explained coffee affects lots of different hormones and processes, not all of which we understand. Ultimately, he believes we should use our common sense.

Dr. Panda says, "If coffee is the last thing in this world that makes you happy, then have it." To which I replied, "Yes, coffee is indeed the last thing in the world that makes me happy."

So yes, drink coffee while fasting, and remember:

■ Coffee you drink while fasting must be black

■ That means no milk, no sugar, and no 400 calorie frappachappachino from Starbucks

Actually, Dr. Panda seemed more concerned about stressing that I shouldn't drink coffee too late in the day. His work is all about optimizing our circadian rhythm, and he reminded me that the half-life of coffee is six hours. Drink a cup of coffee at 4pm and you'll still have half the caffeine in your system at bedtime. So strong early coffees work good for me. Then the food comes later.

DRINK YOUR BRAIN JUICE

Coffee can help with brain meh. It has neuroprotective benefits and the effects from polyphenols and bioactive compounds in coffee are associated with a reduced risk of cognitive decline. Alzheimer's expert Dr. Dale Bredesen says "its stimulant effect increases alertness and cognitive performance and slows memory decline". So you can feel good about being a coffeeholic.

AVOIDING SPIKES AND CRASHES: NO MORE DOUBLE HELPINGS OF APPLE CRUMBLE

We move now from fuel timings to fuel rules. In these days of heightened focus on our health and immunity, it turns out that, of all the things you can do to protect yourself from illness, one important one is to have smaller desserts. It'll massively activate your inner vitality too. Granted, this rule does not seem particularly radical. But there's a radical way of proving to yourself that this is a good idea. Let me explain.

I sought out Dr. Matt Cook to help me with my immunity levels, and his initial recommendation surprised me. It wasn't an exotic supplement or a radical new diet: instead he wanted to emphasize some of the research that identifies the correlation between blood sugar levels and energy. Studies have indicated that diets high in simple carbohydrates may be associated with feelings of fatigue and low energy (10). As he explained, the more you can keep your blood sugar relatively stable, the more you can boost your energy, as well as general health and immunity. That's something that isn't helped by double helpings of apple crumble.

So where is the "radical" part? I love a dessert. I feel pretty healthy. What's the problem?

One of the most welcome health tech innovations of the last few years has been continuous glucose monitors (CGMs) which can help people with diabetes manage their blood sugar levels. And it turns out that the information from these nifty little monitors can help all of us start to learn the individual foods that affect us. They're easy to use. You buy one from a company like Freestyle Libre, and attach the monitor to your arm for two weeks. It doesn't hurt at all. Then you analyze your results with an app like Veri (link in the Meh Directory).

The results can be fascinating. I thought oats were relatively healthy, but was surprised to find out they spike my blood sugar more than the aforementioned apple crumble. Other lessons have been even more remarkable. The most significant is that a good, intense workout on the day of a heavy meal will help blunt my glucose response. I have found this to be consistent, and have even taken to going for a stroll or doing some squats after a carb-heavy dinner.

These revelations surprised me so much, I messaged my friend who is a type 1 diabetic. I said to him,

"A lot of exercise massively seems to regulate my blood sugar levels. Wow, it's an absolute revelation. Why does nobody tell us

this stuff."

He replied,

"Every Type 1 diabetic is told this stuff but speaking for myself I only fully appreciated a lot of it when I got a CGM."

This illustrates the power of the continuous glucose monitor, and what we can all learn from monitoring our blood sugar levels. It's about getting hard data to work out how your body fuels itself. Then you'll avoid spikes and crashes, and activate your best energy levels.

Interesting but useless side note: rum doesn't seem to spike my glucose levels at all. But rum and coke definitely does. I now mix my rum now with peach-flavored sparkling water from Ugly, which is not quite as sweet but works just fine.

EATING LOW HISTAMINE: NO MORE FOOD MEH

For 25 years, I suffered from a dodgy belly. Then I found out about histamine intolerance. This condition is thought to affect up to 15% of people: it means your body creates and holds onto too much histamine, causing a myriad of different issues related to energy.

This is why I recommend that anyone try a low-histamine diet for a few days just to see if it works for them. For me, this has been an absolute game-changer. Within hours of going low histamine, I had more vitality. And over the subsequent weeks and months, things improved dramatically. I was in better shape, had less bloating and had significantly more energy. Bonus: my seasonal allergies started to go away all on their own without the need for over-the-counter medication.

Histamine intolerance can be hard to diagnose as there are so many different ways people can be affected. So look through the list of histamine-related symptoms below, and see if any apply to you. If so, you may suffer from histamine intolerance.

- Gut issues.
- Diarrhea.
- Bloating.
- IBS.
- Nausea.
- Chronic constipation.
- Inflammation.
- Anxiety.
- Shortage of breath.
- Any skin problems.
- Hives.
- Exhaustion.
- Dizziness.
- Constant sneezes.
- Watery eyes.
- Running nose or blocked nose.
- Headache.
- Numbness.
- Sleeping disorders.
- Reduced blood pressure.
- Restless Leg Syndrome.

That is quite the depressing list of meh. Unfortunately, dealing with histamine intolerance needs to come with a health warning all of its own. I've been through so many of these symptoms, from the truly painful to the socially awkward. For example, people regularly used to think I was crying when I had watery, red, itchy eyes. Not a good look.

Histamine intolerance is often quickly improved with just a dietary change and Vitamins B6 and C (11). The dietary part does however mean that some of the most delicious foods out there are out, for now This list of foods is so tantalizing, it often puts people off before they've even tried cutting them out, but don't be disheartened, the idea is that you will start to reintroduce these foods again soon.

Delicious foods that tend to be high in histamine:

■ Chocolate
■ Avocados
■ Cheese
■ Red wine
■ Yogurt
■ Loads of other good stuff

You cut them out for a bit, start to feel better, then add them back in one at a time while monitoring the results. That's the idea. It doesn't mean that you can never have these foods. Only that you start to have more control around them. You'll see from the alcohol section of this book that I haven't given up on all the good stuff.

If you want to start a low-histamine diet, consider taking the quiz on my sister website, The Histamine Intolerance Site (see link in Meh Directory). Then cut out high-histamine foods for three days or more and see if you have more energy. If you feel better, that's an excellent start. Your symptoms might reduce in which case you'll immediately start feeling more healthy. Great news. The next step may be to find a practitioner to help you in his area.

MAGNESIUM: A 2.1% BOOST

We've covered fuel timings and fuel rules, and now we move on to fuel boosters. Ideally, our nutrition will come from food. But sometimes we need an extra kick. We can get this with natural supplements (not pharmaceuticals). This is a common theme that has emerged from my years of looking into nutrition and energy. With natural supplements, we can cherry-pick certain ways to fill in the gaps our diet.

There are some fuel boosters particularly capable of re-energizing and recharging the body, which I've found to be especially helpful and am going to detail here. The usual disclaimer applies—the following is for informational purposes only, and you should run any new regime past your doctor or health practitioner.

I tracked my energy levels for years (yes I know—you're judging me). One of the more effective supplements for extra vitality was magnesium. It increased my daily energy levels by 2.1 percent. Not as big an increase as I had hoped, but definitely noticeable. Magnesium can aid in maintaining heart health, reducing stress levels and (the big one for me) improved sleep at night.

However, it's important to note these scores did not put magnesium supplements in the "magic pill" range. It's not really about looking for magic pills (though they'd be nice), but finding small incremental tweaks that combine to make a big difference to our vitality levels.

LIPOSOMAL GLUTATHIONE: THE SWEET SMELL OF ENERGY

2.1% is fine, but I wanted something a little bit... punchier. So I asked the aforementioned immunity expert Dr. Matt Cook to help.

Dr. Matt's approach is based on using the most non-invasive, natural and integrative ways possible to heal and optimize our health—and, it turns out, swallowing one of the most gut-wrenchingly awful tasting supplements in existence.

One of his main recommendations was glutathione. This is now a cornerstone of my personal quest to boost my immune support. I use a liposomal glutathione (link in Meh Directory). This is a supplement that helps with energy, detox and wellness. It can support a healthy immune system and help with detox. Unfortunately, it tastes horrendous.

As you take it out of the fridge, your nostrils are assailed by a distinct eggy smell. As you flip open the lid, the eggy smell increases to sewer level. As you swallow your glutathione, you have to make sure to remind yourself that this helps with energy, detox and wellness, and that that's why you are experiencing this pong pain.

MERIVA: NO MORE MEH-MORY

Do you forget things easily? Has your memory become more of a meh-mory?

I take Meriva most days. It's a bio-available form of curcumin/turmeric, and it can help with the brain. In fact, Meriva is absorbed an impressive 18 times faster than regular turmeric. Curcumin comes from the turmeric root, and the source of the bright yellow chemical that will dye everything it comes into contact with. It's what gives many curries their yellow color. But you'd have to put a frankly disgusting amount of turmeric in your curry to hit the same amount as there is in these sweet little Meriva capsules.

Health expert Dr. Rhonda Patrick got me onto Meriva: the benefits apparently include better memory. It'll also improve your attention, mood, and decrease your inflammation.

One important question we haven't covered is this: will supplements like Meriva and others affect your quickly? We want these fuel boosters to work synergistically with our fuel rules and fuel timings. We've listed quite a few supplements in this book, but we obviously don't want to be affecting the fasting process if we take them in the morning.

It is generally thought that supplements need not end your intermittent fast, as long as there is no nutritional value to them. What this means it that certain supplements are just fine, but not supplements such as fish oil, which does have a dietary value. That means the latter should be avoided until your fast is over.

BLUE CANNATINE: IS IT TIME TO JOIN THE BLUE TONGUE CLUB

Want more energy on a stressful day? Interested in sharpening your focus and clearing the brain fog?

There is a powerful blue pill that instantly changes the way you feel. No, not Viagra. It helps you with focus and energy, and... turns your tongue blue. In fact, it turns your mouth so blue they call it the "smurf pill".

Blue Cannatine users have reported an increase in mental performance, focus, clarity, energy, effective workouts—and no jitters. It's pretty powerful, and contains a number of strong performance enhancers including nicotine, caffeine, and methylene blue.

So what's it like? Is it safe? What can it do for us?

The active ingredients include Methylene Blue and nicotine, as well as caffeine. it can help with better memory, focus and mood and is proven safe at the dosage level present in Blue Cannatine. And it turns out nicotine isn't as bad for you as you thought (although smoking definitely is.) You can look for nicotine gums or sprays to help with coordination, vigilance, memory and reaction speed. Or use Blue Cannatine, in which the nicotine is at a lower dose than most other supplements.

I took half of one pill an hour ago. Right now I feel a subtle uplift in mood and a little extra focus.

Be warned: if you use this as a Working From Home focus-booster and then jump on a Zoom call, your tongue will be blue and your colleagues will almost certainly notice.

RESVERATROL: LIVE 14 YEARS LONGER BY DOING THIS

We've focused on some instant energy boosters. Now let's up our fuel game by investing in our long-term energy levels.

Dr. David Sinclair is a professor of genetics and one of the world's leading experts on longevity. He runs the aging research lab at Harvard Medical School. He is also somebody who gets seriously excited by genes. He and his team have discovered a set of genes that have turned out to be really important for "controlling the aging process".

They're called sirtuins or SERT enzymes, and they provide the health benefits of fasting, exercise and so on. He has devoted plenty of energy to looking for easy ways to "turn on" this set of genes, and the most potent one he found was in red wine— resveratrol. Unfortunately, there's not enough resveratrol to be found in red wine to make much of a difference. So put that bottle down. It'll have to be a supplement.

Across numerous studies, Dr. Sinclair has observed that high amounts of resveratrol can have a significant effect on aging. In fact, it can make mice seemingly immune to the perils of a Western diet. This shouldn't necessarily be a green light to go straight to the Mcdonald's drive-thru.

He recommends it even more highly if you combine it with intermittent fasting. He also says it might help the cardiovascular system, protect against cancer and diabetes, and has very little downside.

So you are investing in the future, for a longer, healthier, energized life.

The plot thickens, as resveratrol has been shown in studies to inhibit viruses (12), including flu, Epstein-Barr, RSV, and other common viruses. Hmmm. That's pretty relevant right now. In fact, studies show that resveratrol inhibits the MERS coronavirus (13) (not COVID-19, but another coronavirus), and has antiviral properties.

You should apparently buy a source with 98% trans-Resveratrol, not cis-Resveratrol. Take resveratrol in the morning, as it'll help reset your circadian clock and thus potentially boost your REM sleep at night.

Incidentally, Dr. Sinclair told me that if you followed a certain set of recommendations on longevity, you could lengthen your life expectancy by 14 years. Wow. They include avoiding those heavy-duty new airport scanners where you put your hands up (not the ones you simply walk through). He outlined in precise detail the risks to your body of going through the low intensity millimeter waves present in these scanners and how they cause breaks in

DNA. Apparently very low numbers of DNA breaks in mice don't cause cancer, but they do accelerate aging.

It turns out anyone can request a pat-down instead, so that's what I do. To be honest, it does cause some extra check-in stress. I'll regularly find myself taken off to a separate room at Heathrow Airport by a stern official. I probably have to allow an extra quarter of an hour to go through security. But it's all in the name of an extra 14 years, eh?

IV THERAPY: GET A DRIP

This is a particularly radical way to get your fuel boosters. I'm writing this while sitting in a comfy chair at a venue in East London that looks like a cross between a hospital and a trendy bar. There's a large see-through bag hanging above me and a drip feeding into my arm. If you didn't know me, you'd think I was ill. And perhaps I do have a slight winter bug (the perils of having a toddler at nursery). But while it's nothing serious, I'm feeling the need for an extra pick-me-up.

So, I've come for a drip.

This is where the fuel boosters you are taking are 100% intravenously absorbed by your body. They go straight into bloodstream. You sit in a comfy chair, a needle is attached to your arm, and then, drip, drip, drip, the good stuff goes in.

The science is admittedly fairly thin on the ground. One study showed users who received an intravenous cocktail of B and C Vitamins combined with minerals showed improvements in mood, pain levels and quality of life (14). Not everybody is a fan, and some claim there is a significant placebo effect connected to the practice. But whenever I do it, I have a small but noticeable spring in my step afterwards, and that's the goal of this book. So I'm going to carry on with the IV drips.

These establishments are easily found. Search for "IV" or "Drip" in your local area. It should be carried out by an established doctor and there's normally quite a menu to pick from. A good place to start might be a "Myers Cocktail": a potent combination of B vitamins, usually combined with Vitamin C, Zinc and magnesium. These places will often offer "Energy Drips", "Immunity Drips" "Anti-Aging Drips" and even "Hair Health Drips" (for which the ingredients include B Complex, Zinc, Methionine and a whole load of Amino Acids). All delivered straight into your arm.

$$ warning: this is a long way from being the cheapest way in this book to manage your meh, but it does deliver a big jolt of vitality.

FUEL TECH: ESCAPING THE LION

Let's imagine for one moment we are cavemen and cavewomen, chilling by the campfire. It's evening, and we've just chowed down a lovely meal cooked on the fire. But we still have to be ready at all times for an attack, and you never know when it might come. One minute we're basking in that warm post-barbecue feeling (yep, it was caveman BBQ night again). The next, we spot a rustle in the bushes in the corner of our eye. The local lion is on the scene. He's here to gatecrash the party, and we have to run fast. When you go from chilling to escaping the lion, you go from total relaxation to pure stress. For that, you need a resilient heart, and good heart rate variability (HRV).

HRV refers to how consistently our heart beats. We want the variability of our heart rate to be as high as possible, so we can escape the lion at a moment's notice. And HRV can be affected by what we eat and when. An extra caveman burger on the BBQ could potentially be the difference between escaping the lion and being lion supper.

As the Harvard Medical School website puts it: "If one (a person) is in a more relaxed state, the variation between beats is high." That increases how quickly you are able to switch gears, showing more resilience and flexibility. Over the past few decades, research has shown a relationship between low HRV and worsening depression or anxiety. A low HRV is even associated with an increased risk of death and cardiovascular disease" (15).

Our food choices affect our heart health. So let's round off this section by looking at the radical ways in which we can track how our body responds to changes in our diet and meal timings with HRV. What's measured improves, and we can use your own scores as a baseline score to improve health and heart health. We can measure this with readily available health tech that gives us important information which can inform our future fueling choices. For specific health tech wearable options like the Apple Watch, Oura Ring or Whoop Band, head to the MEH-TRICS section.

But what does all of this have to do with diet? As I consult my fairly unscientific research, based on a sample comprising of me and other people I know who wear HRV trackers, I've found that two things count heavily when it comes to improving HRV scores:

1. The size of the evening meal.

2. The timing of the evening meal.

For me, the evening meal needs to be smaller and earlier. That means a higher, "better" HRV score. I'm getting metrics to prove my heart and body are working more effectively in certain scenarios. I can feel it too, with an extra pulsing energy.

To be clear, this is my own research. It's unscientific. But many of my friends and colleagues tracking these metrics have told me they've found similar results which is why I've put this in here. You might be different, but you won't know unless you gather some metrics of your own.

Because of these findings, I can now see how a heavy, late meal negatively impacts the quality of my sleep and how I feel. Sure, it might be the extra glass of wine or second helping of Cote Du Boeuf, but it still leaves me feeling sluggish, and the stats agree. So try making your evening meal earlier and lighter. See how it improves your mood and physical health. And if you are tracking your HRV, you'll have the stats to prove whether or not it works.

While tracking my own HRV, I was also able to discover the following about myself:

- Lower levels of saturated fat in the evening boost my HRV.

- Eating meat in the evening reduces my HRV. (As a committed carnivore it pains me to say this.)

- My best scores ever came during a two-week holiday in the sunshine. Which is as good a nudge as any to reduce stress and prioritize downtime for the sake of resilience, flexibility, mood and health.

Tracking my HRV has allowed me to discover what affects my energy and heart health over time. You might find the complete opposite to me when you start to track your own heart rate. That's the beauty of collecting metrics. Over time, you can pin down what works best for you. Although two weeks on the beach isn't likely to do any harm.

Start tracking the link between fuel, energy and HRV by downloading a free HRV tracking app, or investing in an HRV wearable. There are links in the Meh Directory.

Remember the quality of the fuel you put in your body determines how well it will run. So up your fuel game. Focus on fuel timings, fuel rules and fuel boosters, and start to figure out what works best for you. You'll boost your immune system, be less inflamed, and have more zing.

References

1. Effectiveness of Intermittent Fasting and Time-Restricted Feeding Compared to Continuous Energy Restriction for Weight Loss—https://www.ncbi.nlm.nih.gov/pmc/articles/PMC6836017/

2. Efficacy of fasting and calorie restriction (FCR) on mood and depression among ageing men—https://pubmed.ncbi.nlm.nih.gov/24097021/

3. Safety, health improvement and well-being during a 4 to 21-day fasting period in an observational study including 1422 subjects—https://www.ncbi.nlm.nih.gov/pmc/articles/PMC6314618/

4. Fasting-mimicking diet and markers/risk factors for aging, diabetes, cancer, and cardiovascular disease—https://www.ncbi.nlm.nih.gov/pmc/articles/PMC6816332/

5. Coffee Consumption and Cardiovascular Disease: A Condensed Review of Epidemiological Evidence and Mechanisms—https://pubmed.ncbi.nlm.nih.gov/29276945/

6. Coffee and caffeine intake and incidence of type 2 diabetes mellitus: a meta-analysis of prospective studies—https://pubmed.ncbi.nlm.nih.gov/24150256/

7. Inconsistency of Association between Coffee Consumption and Cognitive Function in Adults and Elderly in a Cross-Sectional Study (ELSA-Brasil)—https://pubmed.ncbi.nlm.nih.gov/26610556/

8. Habitual coffee consumption and risk of cognitive decline/dementia: A systematic review and meta-analysis of prospective cohort studies—https://pubmed.ncbi.nlm.nih.gov/26944757/

9. Human Consumption of Microplastics—https://pubs.acs.org/doi/full/10.1021/acs.est.9b01517

10. The biopsychology of mood and arousal—https://scholar.google.com/scholar_lookup?title=The+biopsychology+of+mood+and+arousal&author=RE+Thayer&publication_year=1989&

11. Histamine and histamine intolerance—https://academic.oup.com/ajcn/article/85/5/1185/4633007

12. Antiviral activity of resveratrol—https://pubmed.ncbi.nlm.nih.gov/20074034/

13. Effective inhibition of MERS-CoV infection by resveratrol—https://pubmed.ncbi.nlm.nih.gov/28193191/

14. Intravenous Micronutrient Therapy (Myers' Cocktail) for Fibromyalgia: A Placebo-Controlled Pilot Study—https://www.ncbi.nlm.nih.gov/pmc/articles/PMC2894814/

15. Heart rate variability: A new way to track well-being—https://www.health.harvard.edu/blog/heart-rate-variability-new-way-track-well-2017112212789

Meh-busting Fuel Reminders...

1

Eat two meals a day. Use intermittent fasting. Avoid snaccidents. Boost your mood. Shrink your waistline.

2

**Follow the Rules of Fuel.
No more puddings or food comas.
Activate deep reserves of energy.**

3

**Try targeted supplements.
For mood, memory, immunity and energy.
Nb: there's no magic pill.**

Chapter Six

Alcohol

" You could drink two bottles of this stuff, and you won't have any hangover whatsoever. **"**

TODD WHITE

Why this theme?

Now we devote a whole section to that most noble of causes: hacking hangovers and staying energized even when drinking alcohol (responsibly, of course).

I am unfortunately Mr. Sensitive these days when it comes to booze. Maybe it's an age thing. Or maybe I always was a lightweight. But just like many people, I still do want the occasional drink. You may do as well.

It turns out there are some unusual, radical hacks you can employ to drink cleaner and feel better the next day. Sure, alcohol can be toxic. But so can oxygen, water and even carrots in the wrong dosage. (Some years ago, an unfortunate death did actually happen due to the overconsumption of carrots.) All this tells us that dosage is everything. When you get your alcohol intake right, a review of the literature shows it can boost your overall happiness, euphoria, and pleasant, carefree feelings (1). Sounds good, right?

Of course, the best way for us all to avoid that hangover feeling is to not drink in the first place. If you've got some meh going on and are also drinking more than a couple of drinks a night or a couple of times a week, you need to cut it down. This is the first lifestyle change you're going to want to make. Get specialist help if you need. Lecture over.

What can you expect in this section?

We're about to cover wine tech (yes that's a thing), supplements that help you deal with hangovers, and the wonderfully named "biodynamic wine". We'll also delve deep into ancient and somewhat forgotten practices for helping the body deal with alcohol.

Using these methods will make you feel better even when you are indulging in the odd glass of something nice. And they'll boost your health and vitality the next day.

CLEAN WINE: TWO BOTTLES AND NO HANGOVER?

"The thing is," my friend Todd said to me, "you can drink two bottles of this stuff, and you won't have any hangover whatsoever tomorrow."

I was at his surprisingly wild party in Austin, Texas. We were sipping on biodynamic wine in the open-plan lounge of one of the coolest houses I'd ever seen. We looked out on a bunch of supposed health nuts going crazy on the dance floor. Over on the sideboard, large platters of ketogenic food were extravagantly piled up. Half-empty bottles of wine lay on every table.

Todd didn't seem remotely concerned that 150 people were getting increasingly out of control. In fact, the entire street outside appeared to be blocked with revelers. No, he was hell-bent on convincing me to down two bottles of wine and see if I had a hangover. Todd believes the world of wine is not well regulated, and that lots of suspicious ingredients can end up making you feel sub-optimal.

Significant efforts have been made to produce healthier organic and sulfite-free wines, and that's where Todd comes in. *Dry Farms Wines* natural wines are low-sulfite, as well as sugar-free and low-alcohol. Todd and his friend David Alred created this company a few years ago and it's now grown into a Goliath of the natural wine world. And—the bit that seals the deal for many—they lab-test all their wines for purity and sulfite levels. They may love a particular bottle of white, for example, but if it doesn't meet the purity test, they will ditch it.

DID YOU KNOW

Wine is not required to have a contents label on the
bottle. There are 76 legal additives approved for use in
winemaking by the US government. This makes it hard
for us to know what's actually in a particular glass of wine.
There might be preservatives, chemicals or coloring
ingredients such as "Mega Purple" to enhance the look
of the wine. Sulfites in wine are also a problem and have
been shown to cause health problems for some people
(2).

So did I drink the two bottles? Almost. Despite being sold on the
company and their tasty natural biodynamic wine, I just couldn't
quite bring myself to finish both. Would I really feel nothing the next
day, I wondered? I sneaked out to my Uber at 2 am as Todd was
uncorking another bottle. I was merry, but not "two-bottles merry".
And the next day I was indeed good to go.

Look up Dry Farm Wines in the Meh Directory, or find a local natural
wine seller. Ask them for their biodynamic range and look for
organic, low-sugar, low-sulfite wines. Avoid the badditives and start
to explore a new way of enjoying wine.

Side note: My first date with my wife was at a brilliant biodynamic
wine bar in London called Terroir. I think it's fair to say it was
a successful venue choice. As a result biodynamic wine has a
particularly special place in my heart.

WINE TECH: A MAGIC WAND

Most of us get some kind of hangover reaction from red wine. Part of the reason for this is that it is mega-high in histamine, sometimes up to 200 times more so than even white wine. Studies show that wine can cause the blood vessels in the brain to dilate, causing wine headaches (3). If only we could wave a magic wand to make that hangover go away.

Enter The Wand. It is described as "A Wine Filter That Removes Histamines & Sulfite Preservatives." With thousands of positive ratings on Amazon, this is something I was keen to know more about. So I put it to the test with a mug of wine (classy I know) that I had opened to use for cooking.

I dunked the wand into the wine for a few minutes, then removed and threw away, and cooked with the wine. It was a delicious French chicken recipe, since you ask, which went down extremely well. But the real test was afterwards. How would I feel? Did I get a wine headache? Did the wine wand work? Could I start to buy the odd bottle of red wine again?

The answer is that... rather, disappointingly, my experiment was not a complete success. Theoretically I should have had minimal headache symptoms after the removal of the histamines and sulfites. I did however still have a bit of a reaction, and my heart rate was still elevated after the red wine. (More in the MEH-TRICS section on quantifying your reactions to things like wine). The results may be different for you.

I haven't given up hope. There is a posh version of the wine wand called Ullo. It also claims to remove sulfites from wine and also has terrific reviews. This is a more high-end product. In the interests of research, I continue to test responsibly as I love to enjoy the very occasional, sensible glass of wine.

Is that so much to ask?

THE WORLD'S CLEANEST VODKA: CUTTING THE PRESERVATIVES, CONGENERS AND IMPURITIES

This section is rapidly becoming a boozefest, so let me just reiterate that I hardly ever drink. It's just special occasions, honest Guv. After all the usual caveats about sensible drinking have been applied, we've established that we may still want the occasional tipple. And I might have cracked it with this fave voddie.

As we've already seen, the idea is that the less additives, preservatives, or impurities there are in an alcohol, the less likely it might be to give you a stinking three-day hangover.

On my quest for clean booze, somebody suggested I try Tito's Handmade Vodka.

It's a product American readers may well be a lot more familiar with than readers in the UK. It is micro-distilled six times in an old-fashioned pot, and is described as "a spectacularly clean product of incomparable excellence". Only the heart of the run ("the nectar") is taken, and the vodka is cleansed of phenols, esters, congeners, and organic acids by filtering it through the finest activated carbon available. Theoretically, removing all these nasties should give you more energy after drinking it moderately. It's also certified gluten-free, which many alcohols are not.

In the name of feeling good the next day, it's worth seeking out brands which make a special effort to provide clean alcohol. It may or may not work, but cleaner vodka does help me. Well, it doesn't give me the night sweats after drinking it, at least.

TOTALLY USELESS—BUT FUN—NLP TECHNIQUE

I have a friend who has an impressive biodynamic wine collection at home. He recently came over to dinner, and brought a posh-looking bottle. I asked him teasingly if he'd lazily taken it out of his collection, rather than purchasing some decent wine especially for the occasion. He said, "of course not, Tony, I bought it on the way here. It was one of the most expensive bottles too." As he did this, I looked very closely at where his eyes went.

NLP eye-accessing cues tell us that, as a rule, as you look at someone, they will look to the right when they're remembering something. And they will look to the left when they're imagining something. This occurs with nearly all right-handers and some left-handers. My friend said he'd stopped at our local supermarket to buy the wine as he very clearly looked upwards and to the left. That told me he was telling a fib, as he laughingly confessed.

This knowledge won't help specifically with energy. It's just fun to know. And it also means I've successfully managed to get an NLP tip in this otherwise biohack-packed section.

ACTIVATED CHARCOAL: HOW COULD EATING DIRT POSSIBLY HELP?

Charcoal has been used for thousands of years to help people who are suspected of having been poisoned, but the first reported use of it as an antidote occurred in 1811. French chemist Michel Bertrand embarked on a bold experiment in which he would consume a lethal amount of arsenic—150 times the lethal dose—and then take charcoal afterwards. He survived (4).

Charcoal binds to toxins and helps get rid of them. Which is kind of useful when you've poisoned yourself in the name of research.

Head down to your local health food shop these days, and you might find some kind of trendy charcoal, honey and menthol remedy shot. Yes, charcoal is definitely "in", and perhaps with good reason. It is a super absorber. It binds to toxins and helps eliminate them, which will help with your energy levels afterwards.

Charcoal is a bit of a miracle cure for me, and not just when it comes to alcohol. There is nothing that can deplete my energy quicker than when I have a stomach ache, or I'm feeling a little bit nauseous or under the weather. When this happens, activated charcoal is not far off a panacea. I carry it around in my backpack in London just in case, and I never go on holiday without some in my suitcase. It really is that powerful. The science backs up my just-in-case-luggage-packing system. In a double-blind, randomized study, symptoms of bloating and abdominal cramps were significantly reduced in groups from two separate countries with activated charcoal (5).

You want to buy good quality activated charcoal tablets. See the Meh Directory for my recommendations. Some say you should take a tablet in between every alcoholic drink, and others simply recommend having them when you've finished—like before you go to bed. Experiment and see what works most effectively for you. And make sure you take them away from other supplements, as they can absorb the nutrients you were expecting to get from those other pills too.

So drink moderately, intersperse with charcoal and plenty of water, and you might have more bounce afterwards.

DAO SUPPLEMENTS: FOUR-PILLS-IN-ONE, ALL IN THE NAME OF A HANGOVER

There is an odd four-pills-in-one supplement in a transparent shell, called a DAO supplement. You can see the four pills rattling around in their cage. And it's effective enough that I will check if I have it in my coat pocket before I go out for a rich meal and a couple of drinks.

This supplement works by focusing on DAO, the primary enzyme that degrades ingested histamine. Remember that histamine plus wine often equals meh. It also contains Vitamin C and Quercetin. My experience with it is positive. Last night, I ate quite a high-histamine meal, with alcohol. I took a DAO supplement before I ate, and today I feel good: no reactions. Bonus.

Here are some potential benefits of taking a DAO supplement:

- It helps to support inflammatory responses in your digestive tract.

- It can boost digestion and metabolism

- It is a good source of the diamine oxidase (DAO) enzyme

Note: This is an effective supplement. However, in the past I haven't recommended it, solely because of the ingredients used in almost every brand on the market. Most of them contain talc (or hydrated magnesium silicate to give it the official title). Talc is added to supplements for all sorts of reasons and, as a food additive, it is "generally recognized as safe" by the FDA. That said, there are numerous experts who don't believe that it is a great ingredient to be including in a supplement. One study suggests no indication for gene toxicity or developmental toxicity. However further research is recommended (6).

So I'll leave you to decide on the validity of hydrated magnesium silicate in a supplement, but thankfully, there are now one or two brands that are talc free. They include the brand I take, DAOfood Plus: again, there's a link in the Meh Directory.

This is a cheap way to mitigate the effects of hangovers and make the odd alcoholic drink a perfectly energizing option. Collect your own metrics to see if this is something you should take regularly

DHM: THE JAPANESE RAISIN TREE

Hovenia Dulcis (or the Japanese raisin tree) is a deciduous tree with alternate, heart-shaped or oval leaves. And it might be about to help you with your next stinking hangover.

The fruit, stalks and flesh of the raisin tree have been used for thousands of years. It appeared as an anti-hangover remedy in China's first pharmacopeia dating back to the 7th century. But here in the West we are only just starting to catch up. Hovenia Dulcis or Semen Hoveniae extracts (don't be put off by the name) have been shown to relieve alcohol toxicity, prevent drunkenness and protect against alcohol-induced liver injuries (7, 8).

Those leaves provide the catchily-titled Dihydromyricetin—which is a mouthful. So let's call it DHM. It's natural, herbal, and available in supplement form. You can pop it during and after you drink to help with your hangover. Don't forget to drink a lot of water as well.

It works by speeding up your liver's ability to metabolize alcohol. This allows your liver to get back to normal more quickly and lessens the damage that the alcohol has done. That's the reason it's so popular all over Japan. Processing alcohol faster means feeling better and bouncier more quickly. You can thus expect to feel significantly perkier the next day.

One significant snag is that DHM is not actually sold in every country. It's not even licensed in some. The nature of biohacking is that we do our own research on products and supplements (using metrics to help), and make our own decisions on what to use.

Also bear in mind that, if you don't fancy harnessing the power of the raisin tree, or are unable to, positive effects have also been observed with the humble milk thistle.

References

1. The psychological benefits of moderate alcohol consumption: a review of the literature—https://pubmed.ncbi.nlm.nih.gov/4053968/

2. Resveratrol: A Fair Race Towards Replacing Sulfites in Wines—https://www.ncbi.nlm.nih.gov/pmc/articles/PMC7288175/

3. Wine and headache—https://pubmed.ncbi.nlm.nih.gov/8645981/

4. Activated charcoal for acute overdose: a reappraisal—https://www.ncbi.nlm.nih.gov/pmc/articles/PMC4767212/#bcp12793-bib-0003

5. Efficacy of activated charcoal in reducing intestinal gas: a double-blind clinical trial—https://pubmed.ncbi.nlm.nih.gov/3521259/

6. Re-evaluation of calcium silicate (E 552), magnesium silicate (E 553a(i)), magnesium trisilicate (E 553a(ii)) and talc (E 553b) as food additives—https://www.ncbi.nlm.nih.gov/pmc/articles/PMC7009349/

7. Influence of Hovenia dulcis on alcohol concentration in blood and activity of alcohol dehydrogenase (ADH) of animals after drinking—https://pubmed.ncbi.nlm.nih.gov/17048612/

8. Semen Hoveniae extract protects against acute alcohol-induced liver injury in mice—https://pubmed.ncbi.nlm.nih.gov/20673184/

Meh-busting Alcohol Reminders...

1

Drink clean. Choose pure, lab-tested alcohols to minimize hangovers. Avoid "badditives". Dose carefully.

2

Eat dirt. Activated charcoal binds to toxins and helps get rid of them. Take before drinking and after.

3

The DAO of life. The DAO enzyme degrades ingested histamine. Take a DAO supplement before a glass of something nice.

Chapter Seven

Home

"

Ah! There is nothing like staying at home, for real comfort.

"

JANE AUSTEN

Why this theme?

If you want more energy, you need to tackle "meh" where you live. Our home should be a sanctuary—a place to retreat, relax and escape. The more that you can recharge your battery in your home environment, the more you can re-emerge into the world at 100%.

So we're going to make some easy, energizing alterations aimed at optimizing your living space, so your energy goes through the roof.

What can you expect in this section?

The area of biohacking leans on primal principles. It learns from the best of what worked for our ancestors. And it adapts them to create some extraordinary ideas for boosting the comfort of our home. We'll make it non-toxic, low-EMF, more primal, and clutter-free. Sometimes we'll employ tech, and other times our solutions will be radically simple. We'll take a look at our:

- Kitchen

- Bedroom

- Bathroom

- Home Office

- And even closet

That way, when we step out of our front door, we can re-emerge into the world fully fired up and ready to go.

WATER FILTER: THE RED FOOD DYE TEST

Dehydration leads to meh. It affects our body and our cognitive performance. (1) With this first home hack, you can make sure that the water you're drinking to hydrate is clean and boosts your energy efficiently.

We are lucky to live at a time when the water that comes into our homes has been treated to get rid of bad bacteria, parasites, and other nasty organisms. But the chemicals that treat water are not necessarily optimal for our physiology. The water we generally presume to be clean can be affected by treatment that was intended to remove contaminants and other harmful byproducts (2).

So we want to prioritize good, clean water for the optimal running of our brain and body. I recommend that you invest in a good filter.

There are many water filters on the market, including filter jugs, filter bottles and filter taps from all sorts of companies. You can buy them in the supermarket, local hardware store and online. But not all filters are created equal. I'm an evangelist for the Berkey water filter. It sits on your countertop, and can remove chlorine and chloramine (used for water disinfection), viruses, harmful pathogenic bacteria, cysts, heavy metals, parasites and hazardous chemicals, while keeping in the essential minerals you need.

Calling any filtered water "delicious" might be a bit of a stretch, but it does taste good and inspire me to hydrate more regularly.

Here's an impressive test you can perform on my favorite filter: you can pour a full bottle of red food dye into the upper chamber, and the filter will take it all out as it trickles through to the lower chamber. If any comes through, it means you haven't assembled it properly. Many worry about pharmaceuticals in our water supply:

it also removes 99.5% of those. And if you live in an area where fluoride is added to the water, it has an optional add-on that can remove that too.

TAP TIP

Preppers are people who prepare for worst-case scenarios like natural disasters: they love Berkey Filters too. In emergencies they can purify raw, untreated water, and have been found to remove 99.9999999% of pathogenic bacteria and 99.999% of viruses. So if the taps stop working, your filter can carrying on providing you with water.

Hopefully it won't come to that, eh?

Water tech is developing all the time, and a cheaper option is the LARQ bottle. This uses UV light to clean and sterilize rather than filtering the water.

If you make the switch from tap water to filtered, I can't honestly say that you'll immediately start walking around with 50% more spring in your step. It's not that kind of method. What you will notice is an improved taste and a cleaner water supply in your home. In other words, it is a long-term investment in being healthier and more energized.

CLEANER AIR: THE WORLD'S FRESHEST AIR

The World Health Organization (WHO) has listed air quality as the single biggest environmental threat to public health. The air we breathe is directly linked to our health. Poor quality air is consistently linked to a laundry-list of health complaints (3). But what about our mood?

Can cleaner air make us feel less meh?

If boosting our happiness and our emotional well-being counts (4) as managing meh, then cleaner air works. In the longer term, air pollution significantly raises the risk of infertility (5). And while most of us think that air pollution is something that happens outside, 90% of our time is, on average, spent indoors. The air we breathe inside is often even worse. It can be up to five times more polluted with mold, chemical gases, carpet fibers, dust, bacteria, viruses, pollution and toxins from overcooked food (a big one).

So how do we clean the air in our homes? Your two options are:

1. Go primitive, and use the German tradition of luften.

2. Get a state-of-the-art air purifier.

Both actually work quite well.

Option 1 basically means opening a window. I told you it was primitive. Luften is basically a word for the German national obsession with room ventilation. It is such a part of the national fabric that luften is regularly observed in schools and homes— opening a window to let in some lovely fresh air. German rental agreements apparently often specify that a home should be aired twice a day. While the rest of the world is sitting toasty in the warmth, the Germans have a window open. And the air they are breathing may well be cleaner as a result.

Admittedly, this is a rudimentary biohack and, if you live by a busy road, luften won't help with the traffic pollution. So, it may be time to go more high-tech with Option 2.

I use a HypoAir Air Angel. The technology was originally developed by NASA and, astonishingly, the research shows that it kills 99% of allergens, odors, germs, and viruses, including various forms of coronavirus. It was even tested on SARS-CoV-2 (the COVID-19 virus) and was found to kill it on a surface outside the unit.

I use one mainly in my bedroom, and I have noticed a difference in my overnight stuffy nose levels (another technical term). My sleep has improved considerably. The first time I used it, I felt like I'd been inhaling lovely cool forest air all night. That meant I felt livelier the following day. I also noticed that being close to certain heaters/radiators in my house makes me feel suboptimal. It's kind of like a heavy headache, and I can't really explain why it happens. However, when I open a window or plug in the purifier, that headache meh dissipates.

STANDING DESKS: STAND UP FOR ENERGY

Let's hack your home office. There is compelling meh-busting research around standing up when you work. In one seven-week study, those using standing desks reported less stress and fatigue (or meh) than those who sat down for the whole day. The clincher is that, when they reverted back to their original desks, their overall mood returned to their previous levels (6).

So, home desk workers of the world, is it time to stand up?

It's cheaper than you think. You can almost certainly adapt your home to stand at your desk for free. There are plenty of ideas online on how to achieve this without spending anything. A convenient shelf and a pile of books will do the trick. There's even an inventive blogger who built a standing desk using a chopping board, two wooden salad bowls, a tension curtain rod, and a copy of the Oxford English Dictionary (7).

DESK BREAK

Been working at your standing desk too long? Working from home brings big benefits but it also means that we stare at screens more than ever. Let's switch off for a few moments. This "20/20" hack combines an extremely simple NLP technique for recalibrating the senses with the American Optometric Association's recommendations for dealing with digital eye strain.

1. Step away from the desk. You might be standing but you still need to take a break.

2. Look out of the window at something 20 yards away— the optimum distance to give your eyes a rest.

3. Focus for 20 seconds. Notice colors, brightness and movement. Focus solely on this.

4. Every time your mind wanders, start the 20 seconds again. It may be surprising how many times you have to start the 20 seconds again.

By paying attention to your attention span, you take a moment to reconnect. It gives your brain and your eyes a chance to refocus before you come back to your desk.

I'm writing this now at a standing desk. I don't stand all day: instead, I alternate between standing and sitting. It allows me more movement throughout the day and feels better on my back.

This is a clear continuation of the GOYAP (Getting Off Your Ass Program) we encountered in the EXERCISE section. It's exactly what we are looking for in this book—simple changes that make a big difference. You'll feel healthier and happier when you work standing up. All for the price of two salad bowls and a dictionary.

PRESSURE COOKER: ONE KITCHEN GADGET TO RULE THEM ALL

It's thought microwaves take lot of the nutrients out of food. They have been found, for example, to remove 97% of the flavonoids—ie the good stuff—in broccoli (8). So it was a particularly satisfying day when I threw the microwave in the dump and said goodbye to Frankenfood forever.

It was a pressure cooker that made it possible. It is the most impressive bit of kitchen tech I've ever owned, and it gets used almost every day. It's healthy and quick. It cooks, steams, sautés, makes yogurts, and so much more.

It's so handy I'm in danger of becoming a pressure cooker bore. I use an Instant Pot. It's particularly good for histamine levels. You can cook frozen food quickly and safely in it. You'll get that "slow-cooked" taste to food without actually having to leave it in a slow cooker for 10 hours where it would accumulate too much histamine.

My favorite dishes:

- Bulletproof Beef Shin (inspired by the Bulletproof Cookbook—link in Meh Directory) with olive oil, turmeric, and other spices. I cook from frozen for even more freshness and the pressure cooker deals with it perfectly. Put in the pot for 1 hour and 15 minutes. Then shred with a tablespoon of Apple Cider Vinegar, which is the secret ingredient. Any leftover liquid goes in the freezer for a stock for the dish below.

- ▥ "Beau Rice": put on sauté mode for bacon, onions, and garlic, then the rice goes in with chopped veggies and spices for 12 minutes. A perfect easy dinner. It can be made as a lower carb meal without rice and with more chopped cauliflower and sweet potato. Then it's just five minutes to cook.

- ▥ Low Histamine Yogurt. This is a work in progress, and has involved a number of disgusting yogurt failures. However it is a lot of fun to try the yogurt mode.

Upgrading your kitchen like this will help with our ultimate goal. You'll be able to eat well and feel energized afterwards.

BATHROOM CABINET UPGRADES: ENERGY BOOSTS IN SURPRISING PLACES

Surely we can't upgrade your energy levels in the bathroom? Yes we can... starting with toothpaste. This one might seem crazy, as so many people don't know about it. There is an ingredient known as a synthetic detergent in toothpaste that causes many people to get mouth ulcers. It's called Sodium Lauryl Sulfate or SLS. If you have mouth ulcers then when you switch toothpaste, you might find that they magically go away.

That's what happened to me. I used to get loads of them until I switched to natural toothpaste. It's not just hearsay—there's science to this too. Norwegian researchers found that patients brushing with a "detergent-free placebo paste" had a significantly lower frequency of mouth ulcers. Oral health and an overall sense of health and well-being are interlinked ,so expect to feel better both now and in the long term (9).

- Bathroom energy booster 1. Try using a natural toothpaste without SLS and see if your irritating mouth ulcers go away. Energy win if they do.

Now let's look at some of the other personal care products you use. Where do toxins come from? Well, they can be hiding in your food, your home, the phone in your pocket, or even the shampoo you use. They can lurk in the moldy corner of a basement, in a cheap plastic water bottle, or in your bathroom cabinet. Regardless of where they are hiding, they could be having a big impact on your day-to-day vitality levels as well as potentially causing serious long-term health issues (10, 11).

You have two options here. You could read every ingredient on every bottle in every room in your house and bathroom cabinet. Then google each ingredient separately and see if there appears to be any harmful ingredients. You'd be looking for the likes of; BHA and BHT, P-phenylenediamine, DEA-related ingredients, Dibutyl phthalate, Formaldehyde-releasing preservatives, Parabens, Parfum (sometimes known as simply fragrance), Petrolatum, Siloxanes, Sodium Lauryl Sulfate (our old friend), and Triclosan.

Trust me, this is not an efficient use of your time.

Or you could free up some headspace, and use an app that does it all for you.

There are quite a few apps out there that can help in this area. *Think Dirty* is outstanding. Scan the stuff in your bathroom cabinet, and get color-coded science and research on the ingredients. You might be surprised at how many supposedly "natural" products show up as irritants or toxic. As a result of learning some of these dirty little skin secrets, I've changed to a number of cleaner options. EWG's Skin Deep site does something similar.

- Bathroom Energy Booster 2: Clean out the toxic beauty products and fragrances from your bathroom cabinet. Protect your energy now and in the future.

One product I found really helpful to learn more about was sunscreen. We absorb 60% of what we put on our skin into our bloodstream, so slathering sunscreen all over means any potential irritants go straight in. That's not good for our long-term vitality. Unfortunately, many "clean" sunscreens have a rather white, chalky appearance. However, it is possible to pursue the Love Island tan without the wrinkles. After exhaustive testing, I've found slightly tinted ones to be most effective in terms of spreadability, sunburn protection and social acceptability. My favorite is listed in the Meh Directory.

There's time for one more foray into the bathroom cabinet. On my journey to find more vitality, I've tried the good, the bad, and the utterly bonkers. This next detox method falls in the third camp. However, in the interest of being transparent about the energy methods that do and don't work, I'm going to tell you about it anyway.

My friend Dr. Steve Simpson is a mind coach who works with some of the world's top poker players. As a medical doctor, he has a real interest in how the mind and the body can work as healthily as possible together. That means his poker players and other sports stars get to operate at their best. And he will work on anything from mind games to bathroom accessories to help them achieve that.

One day, he told me a story that intrigued me. He'd known a man for many years who was renowned in the local community for being a miserable so-and-so. He was particularly grumpy. It was nothing personal: he was just like that with everybody. So when Dr. Steve turned up at a lunch and discovered he was sitting next to him, he steeled himself for a long couple of hours. But—surprise, surprise— his neighbor turned out to be the life and soul of the party. In the past, Mr. Grumpy would have been obnoxious. He would have complained about everything from politics to the food. This time though, he was in backslappingly good form.

All the other guests were amazed by this transformation. When he went to the bathroom, they decided they had to delicately ask him what had happened. But they had to do this tactfully, without making it obvious how much they preferred the new version. He bounced back from the bathroom and somebody plucked up the courage to ask him. They said, "You're in good form. Have you been taking any magic pills from the doctor?".

He laughed. "No." He paused for a moment, and then continued. "As a matter of fact, though, I have been doing something different. Over the past couple of months, I've been using some footpads I bought online. They draw the toxins out of the skin through your feet."

Dr. Steve asked, "And how does it make you feel?"

He replied, "It makes me feel happy. I can't explain why, but I've never felt as happy as this."

At this point—obviously—all the other guests round the table immediately asked him where they could buy these footpads.

Dr. Steve and I did exactly the same thing; we went on Amazon to buy some. We found a surprising selection of choices for detox foot pads. The idea is that you apply them to the soles of your feet at night. They supposedly "draw the toxins out of the skin." Some of them even carry a warning that you shouldn't touch the pads in the morning because the toxins that come out will be black: and if you get black goo, that is apparently particularly toxic. They are natural products that use bamboo vinegar along with ginger, lavender, wormwood and green tea to draw out the bad stuff (who knew). We were intrigued.

We conducted our own little investigation. But we unfortunately found that, although it's a great story, there really isn't much in the way of science to back up these footpads. Yes, they make your feet black in the morning, but they certainly didn't turn out to be life-changing for us.

■ Bathroom Energy Booster 3: Try detox foot pads but with a healthy dose of skepticism. Maybe they'll energize you or maybe they won't, but it's fun to try this stuff out and very inexpensive.

One of the things I like about my energy adventure, is that sometimes you come across something so gloriously crazy there is no rational sense to it. Black goo coming out of the feet isn't for me, but it still seems to work for some people. It clearly worked for Mr. Grumpy. And, judging by the impressive reviews online, it works for thousands of others. I'm all in favor of effective detox, but, to me, the footpads are not as important as cleaning up the products you use on a day-to-day basis.

AVOIDING EMFS: IS THAT A PHONE IN YOUR POCKET OR ARE YOU JUST HAPPY TO SEE ME?

How much should we worry about electromagnetic fields (EMFs), mobile signals, and Wi-Fi in our home?

They are, unfortunately, pretty much all over the place. They come from the ever-increasing amount of tech we accumulate. That means every device that sends or receives signals like Wi-Fi or a cell phone signal. And there are some good reasons why you might want to think about reducing the EMFs in your home.

1. Some people experience an immediate difference in their energy levels when they cut the EMFs. Some studies suggest that EMF exposure affects sleep and mood (12), although other scientists have argued that the evidence is weak.

2. Are EMFs affecting us in the long term? Research shows that the adverse effects of exposure from cell phones and other wireless transmitting devices include increased rates of cancer, chromosomal DNA damage, impaired brain development in children, and fertility issues (13). The study concludes, "having a cell phone next to the body is harmful" In addition, the World Health Organization says that mobile phone radiation is "possibly carcinogenic".

3. Consider the sheer range of devices we own that emit a signal. Wi-Fi routers, cell phones, laptops, games consoles, thermostats, radios, TVs and more are all combining to an invisible and potentially damaging "EMF soup".

EMFs and Cell Phones

Let's start by protecting your most sensitive area. If you are like me, your phone spends a lot of time in your pocket. There are some compelling (though inconclusive) studies on EMF radiation from devices like phones. The same study I mentioned above suggests that men who keep cell phones in their trouser pockets have significantly lower sperm counts and significantly impaired sperm motility (the ability for sperm to swim correctly) and morphology. Shudder. I should emphasize that not everybody thinks EMFs, Wi-Fi, and mobile signals are worth worrying about.

There are plenty of methods for mitigating their effects. Here are a few free options.

▨ Don't put your phone in your pocket, or touch it to your ear.

▨ Use airplane mode liberally when your phone is in your pocket.

It's hard to remember to always use these free options. So you can also make use of other affordable options;

▨ Get an EMF-blocking laptop pad.

▨ Use a mobile phone case which deflects the signal away from your most sensitive area.

If you need some ideas, the Gadget Guard case is snappily described as "the world's only case with patented technology proven to reduce cell phone radiation by up to 75% while maintaining signal strength." And SafeSleeve provides protection on your phone while you're holding it to your ear. There are links in the Meh Directory.

You may or may not feel an instant energy boost from addressing this issue. But the research suggests you'll be protecting your health and energy long-term.

EMFs and headphones

From your crown jewels to your brain,... low-EMF tech has extended to headphones too.

As you stroll around the neighborhood talking to your friends on your fancy Bluetooth earphones, has it occurred to you that these also conduct a signal close to your brain? This might be especially important for children, whose developing brains are vulnerable to electromagnetic radiation (14).

So, what to do?

You could swap out the Bluetooth or wired headphones for hollow air tubes. These conduct the sound to your ears via sound waves using no metal. These tubes replace the traditional wires found inside Bluetooth headphones and can cut the radiation by up to 99% compared to normal phone use. I'd love to recommend these. Unfortunately, the sound from every pair I've ever used is tinny, and the design is flimsy. That makes me feel more meh, not less! Maybe you'll find them more bearable.

If you are one of those people sensitive to EMFs, using air tubes may well improve your energy instantly. Just don't expect your music to sound good. Air tubes are not a perfect listening experience. It's one area where the EMF-friendly tech is yet to catch up.

EMFs and, er, Underwear

We are now getting into one of the most gloriously bonkers parts of this book.

I have a delightful pair of boxer shorts that block wireless radiation. Who knew such a thing existed? They use silver-lining technology that has been tested and certified to block over 99% of cell phone and Wi-Fi radiation. Yet, somehow, they feel surprisingly normal to wear.

The company is called Lambs: they are fond of quoting a US government peer review study from 2018. It concluded that there is "clear evidence" that radiation from mobile phones causes cancer (15). This is important as, in this section of the book, we are looking to preserve both our short-term energy and long-term vitality.

If you are interested in boosting your fertility, this is something you may want to look into further, as well as, of course, keeping your phone out of your pocket in the first place. But be prepared to pay considerably more than your normal underwear for the privilege.

EMFs and the family

I've been lucky enough to become a parent recently. It's been an absolute rollercoaster ride so far, and I have loved every minute. Well, apart from the odd 2 am poonami.

In the interests of having a healthy, happy, thriving baby, I wanted the best and most natural home environment. And, as you might expect from reading this book, I spent a long time getting this right. In fact, I wrote a detailed blog on my website just for new parents. If you read it, you'll probably think "this man has far too much time on his hands."

One way you can make a real difference in this area is through your baby monitor. This is something that your little cherub is going to spend a lot of time around. And as we've seen, this can have an impact on energy and health.

In order to communicate without any wires, all baby monitors transmit a signal. Often this signal is really quite strong—which is not good for baby. Most baby monitors, in fact, are constantly emitting radio frequency radiation either in the FM band or as microwaves, all while they are close to baby.

So, the hunt was on for a baby monitor that worked. Trust me, I've read a thousand baby monitor reviews so you don't have to. The winner is Hartig & Helling, who make an "extremely low-radiation" baby monitor which works through a very low analogue radio signal that is voice-activated (important). These radio signals are considered to be safer than the newer digital frequencies (Bluetooth, Wi-Fi, etc). Even the charging units for this monitor are low-EMF. You wouldn't call them hi-tech, but they do the job and protect your baby, And that's all that matters.

All of these solutions based around the issue of EMF may well boost your energy levels immediately, or at least look after you and your family long-term. And you can dive even deeper—my friend Rich has an EMF canopy. He hangs it over his bed at night like an exotic, high-tech mosquito net to block the EMFs from a nearby train station: he loves it so much he even takes it on holiday. There is much debate about how much we feel the effects of EMF in the short and long term, but I do believe the science I've linked to is sufficiently concerning to warrant action.

DEALING WITH THE "TECH TOXINS" IN YOUR HOME: A $7 SOLUTION

"Tech Toxins" aren't just about the electromagnetic fields swirling around us. A dependency on our screens is clearly a growing problem in other respects. I know this from my own addiction to playing chess on my smartphone at two in the morning. I've kicked the habit now, honest.

Anybody who watched the viral hit documentary *The Social Dilemma* on Netflix will know a little about how pervasive the problems of tech and screentime are.

You'll be pleased to hear that I'm not recommending a kitchen safe where you "lock away temptation" overnight. (This was featured in the documentary—but it seems a recipe for disaster). However, we have invested in a $7 (£5) plug timer on the Wi-Fi. That means that, at night, it simply clicks off. No more EMFs from the Wi-Fi overnight, and no more Wi-Fi-based distraction—for anyone in the family—when we should be asleep.

Search for "plug timer" and you'll find one that suits. It is a decidedly lo-fi hack that means better sleep, and more energy the next day.

INFRARED SAUNA: ESCAPE THE BLEAK MEH-WINTER

Back in the lockdown days, I suffered a minor injury: putting my back out. Okay, by the standards of lockdown hardships, this really wasn't that bad, but I was still forced to rethink my "putting the baby in the cot" game. Back injuries can cause huge physical distress as well as, frankly, doing your head in. Luckily, I had the perfect way to sort it out, with something that not everybody is lucky enough to have in their back garden. An infrared sauna.

This is something that has the potential to turn your meh upside down. Infrared heat doesn't just work for your back. It's relaxing while you're in there and energizing once you emerge. It's good for detox, skin and more. There is an increasing body of evidence that suggests saunas of some description are one of the best hacks for short-term mood elevation (16, 17). The research is also impressive when it focuses on longevity and heart health (18).

This home hack is definitely in the "eye-wateringly expensive but worth it" category. And happily, you don't have to do it at home. There are plenty of places you can book in for an hour or more of heat. That way you can escape the bleak midwinter weather, recharge, relax and heal at the same time.

For me, the heat has been a faithful friend during times of low energy or apathy. It was pretty amazing how quickly my back got better. I follow a specific routine: first, stretch a lot, then whack the sauna up high on *pain relief mode*. Half an hour later I would feel considerably looser. Two interesting side notes are my heart rate variability (HRV) stats tend to curve up after use (good news) and I tend to sleep more deeply afterwards (even better news).

Make sure you use a low-EMF infrared sauna like a Sunlighten Sauna (see link in Meh Directory) for all the reasons already listed. Beware cheap imitations which are basically a little bit like microwaving yourself. One more affordable option worth looking at is an infrared sauna blanket like the one sold by Higher Dose. You lie down with the blanket over you and it heats you up in a similar way.

Notice how much more energized you feel during and after your infrared heat experience: for some people this will be one of your best re-energizing methods.

ONE IN, ONE OUT. STAYING CLUTTER-FREE

Many of us spend more time at home than ever before. But our homes aren't fit for this purpose. They haven't caught up. We're trying to work, play, exercise, and sleep within four walls that weren't designed to fulfil so many functions. So, we need to make some of the changes in this section. But we want to be as mindful as possible during this process. Some of them might involve acquiring some *stuff*, so I want to reiterate an important value of mine: to declutter and have *less stuff, not more*.

I'm inspired by the author Paolo Coelho. He lives in a huge apartment in Geneva. And he fills it with... nothing. He says, "empty space is my biggest indulgence".

It turns out that having more space and less stuff to worry about is liberating.

For inspiration, I spoke to Bea Johnson, the world-renowned author of *Zero Waste Lifestyle*. Her big themes are as follows: less clutter, more simplicity, look after the environment, save your energy for the things that matter, and (a biggie) save money. She is adamant that having less stuff and a cleaner space makes a huge difference to her life. Her main bit of advice was extremely simple.

Live by the rule of "one in, one out".

She says, "When you get something new, something else has to go. It can be donated, given away, or recycled. It's a nice way to keep the home clutter-free." Personally, I feel calmer, more relaxed and focused when there's not a load of clutter everywhere. Paolo Coelho says he feels, "possessions complicate things". In the same way, I find it strange how things you own require mental bandwidth. I've found it satisfying to pass on unwanted items via places like Facebook Marketplace. I don't ever miss them and I do love the extra space.

Consider some of these questions as you tweak your home:

■ How can you keep your home clutter-free and simple?

▓ How can you help the environment by buying secondhand, and how can you save money at the same time?

▓ How can you employ the "one in, one out" rule? What can go when you bring in, for example, an air purifier or a pressure cooker?

Stay focused on fostering an environment that gives energy, not saps it.

References

1. The Hydration Equation: Update on Water Balance and Cognitive Performance—https://www.ncbi.nlm.nih.gov/pmc/articles/PMC4207053/

2. What are the trends in the quality of drinking water and their effects on human health?—https://www.epa.gov/report-environment/drinking-water

3. Air pollution—https://www.who.int/health-topics/air-pollution#tab=tab_1

4. How Air Pollution Might Be Affecting Your Mood—https://socialsciences.nature.com/posts/43212-how-air-pollution-might-be-affecting-your-mood-our-study-on-air-pollution-and-happiness-in-china

5. Association between exposure to airborne particulate matter less than 2.5 μm and human fecundity in China—https://www.sciencedirect.com/science/article/pii/S0160412020321863

6. Reducing occupational sitting time and improving worker health: the Take-a-Stand Project, 2011—https://pubmed.ncbi.nlm.nih.gov/23057991/

7. How I Built an Ergonomic Adjustable Standing Desk For Free—https://elanmorgan.medium.com/how-i-built-an-ergonomic-adjustable-standing-desk-for-free-76f7a7f4d0a0

8. Effects of domestic cooking on flavonoids in broccoli and calculation of retention factors—https://www.ncbi.nlm.nih.gov/pmc/articles/PMC6407093/

9. Association between toothbrushing and risk factors for cardiovascular disease: a large-scale, cross-sectional Japanese study—https://bmjopen.bmj.com/content/6/1/e009870?utm_source=TrendMD&utm_medium=cpc&utm_campaign=BMJOp_TrendMD-1

10. REDUCING ENVIRONMENTAL CANCER RISK What We Can Do Now—https://deainfo.nci.nih.gov/advisory/pcp/annualReports/pcp08-09rpt/PCP_Report_08-09_508.pdf

11. Nail polish allergy. An important differential diagnosis in contact dermatitis—https://pubmed.ncbi.nlm.nih.gov/9280695/

12. Extremely Low Frequency Electromagnetic Fields Facilitate Vesicle Endocytosis by Increasing Presynaptic Calcium Channel Expression at a Central Synapse—https://www.nature.com/articles/srep21774

13. Risks to Health and Well-Being From Radio-Frequency Radiation Emitted by Cell Phones and Other Wireless Devices—https://www.ncbi.nlm.nih.gov/pmc/articles/PMC6701402/

14. Health effects of electromagnetic fields on children—https://www.e-cep.org/journal/view.php?doi=10.3345/cep.2019.01494

15. https://getlambs.com/pages/a-letter-from-our-ceo

16. Changes in mood state following whole-body hyperthermia—https://pubmed.ncbi.nlm.nih.gov/1607735/

17. The impact of whole-body hyperthermia interventions on mood and depression—are we ready for recommendations for clinical application?—https://pubmed.ncbi.nlm.nih.gov/31159624/

18. What is an infrared sauna? Does it have health benefits?—https://www.mayoclinic.org/healthy-lifestyle/consumer-health/expert-answers/infrared-sauna/faq-20057954

Meh-busting Home Reminders...

1

Live healthier. Stand while you work. Open windows. Purify the air and water.

2

Deal with "tech toxins". Cut EMFs, mobile signals and Wi-Fi. Reduce your dependency on screens.

3

Use "one in, one out". Stay clutter-free as you switch to a non-toxic, super-natural, low-EMF, greener home.

Chapter Eight

Sleep

"Sleep is our recharge function and our reset button... and we all need a reset button sometimes.

SAM OWEN

Why this theme?

You can't have energy without rest. Of all the tweaks and tricks you can look at for more vitality, optimizing your natural sleep cycle might just be the most powerful. Nothing beats a good night's sleep. It's the "master hack".

There is one fascinating study that demonstrates why striving to improve our sleep is so important. A group of scientists set up a field study where a number of participants went camping in the Rocky Mountains. They left the trappings of modern life behind. That didn't just mean their iPhones: they weren't even allowed a torch.

After a few days, researchers found the campers started sleeping longer. They were getting a luxurious ten hours sleep on average, as opposed to the usual seven and a half (1). They were also going to bed two and a half hours earlier on average. And the clincher was that they were significantly more energetic during the day. Why? The campers were being exposed to up to 13 times more natural light than they would have been at home, which helped every aspect of their circadian rhythm. Getting more in tune with nature meant more fizz during the day and way more sleep at night.

What can you expect in this section?

Most of the methods in this book, however powerful, will still be trumped by a good, deep night's sleep. So now we'll focus obsessively on improving it. We'll look at:

■ how to naturally increase melatonin

■ how to get more REM sleep

- how to avoid "blue light" in the evening

- how to banish sleep FOMO

- how to sleep longer and deeper

- A special sleep "unfair advantage"...

The campers got more natural light. They went to bed earlier. And they slept longer. Happily, you don't have to go camping to get a similar effect.

SWITCHING OFF AT NIGHT: A NOT-VERY-RADICAL-SUGGESTION INVOLVING YOUR CELL PHONE

Our Rocky Mountain campers all left their phones at home. Clearly the experiment wouldn't have worked so well if they'd been checking Instagram in the final moments before bed.

Almost 70% of people have been found to check their mobile phones in the last half hour before sleep. And 62% of us check their phone within 15 minutes of waking up (2). This research was conducted more than four years ago, and I suspect that percentage is now even higher. If you are looking to develop an unfair advantage over most other people in life, this is it:

Leave your phone out of the bedroom.

Put it downstairs. Lock it in a cupboard. Throw it out of the window. Do whatever it takes. Just don't leave it where you sleep.

It's weird that this is a radical concept these days, but that's the world we live in. Do this and you will be behaving differently to most other people.

I confess: it took me a long time to kick the habit of cuddling up with my phone. So sad. I know how tough it is, but the rewards will be great. Now, even if I get FOMO pangs in the middle of the night, my phone has been taken out of the equation so I can't do anything about it anyway. The scientist who set up the Rocky Mountains experiment, Kenneth Wright, said this:

"Living in our modern environments can significantly delay our circadian timing and late circadian timing is associated with many health consequences."

Other research shows an association between poor sleep quality and using your mobile for at least 30 minutes before trying to sleep (after the room lights have been turned off) and between poor sleep quality and having the mobile near your pillow (3, 4).

You'll get an extra advantage the next day too. I sought out Julie Morgenstern, author of the book *Never Check Email in The Morning*. She says when the first thing you look at is your phone, you are setting yourself up for a distracted day. "You'll never recover," she says. "Those requests and those interruptions and those unexpected surprises and those reminders and problems are endless."

Excessive distraction in the morning can affect the brain's ability to perform tasks and do deep work, just when you want it to be at its sharpest.

I seem to go into problem-solving mode more effectively without screens in the bedroom. I wake up with the solutions to problems and a clearer head. I'm in a better mood. It all adds up to an unfair advantage over the sleepy scrollers.

So we're going to improve our sleep and our morning edge. Here's the plan:

1. Set up your bedroom with everything that your phone might provide—alarm clock, book, light, etc.

2. Disinvite your phone from your bedroom, and then maybe...

3. Keep a pen and paper by your bed for any extra inspiration and creativity that might pop up.

At the cost of a little less night-scrolling, you'll be setting yourself up for better sleep, and more energy and creativity the next day.

THE COLOR BLUE: THE REASON NETFLIX MESSES WITH YOUR SLEEP

Bright light at night impacts our sleep. That's perhaps the best of a long list of reasons why watching Netflix at 1am might not be a good idea. It is not just because the latest episode might be so good that you can't switch it off. Although, that is relevant too. It turns out that some of the bright lights we have in our homes and on our devices late at night impact the depth of our sleep, and our long-term health, by suppressing our melatonin levels (5).

This light is known as "blue light", even though it might not be blue to the naked eye. Our bodies respond to this bright blue light by thinking it's daylight. "Woohoo", your body thinks, "look at all this bright light. It must be the middle of the day". Obviously not good for sleep.

The Director of Sleep Medicine at Harvard says, "The more research we do, the more evidence we have that excess artificial light at night can have a profound, deleterious effect on many aspects of human health" (6). And a new study shows nighttime smartphone use damages sperm too. Researchers showed that men who reported using their phone more in the evenings had a reduced concentration of sperm, as well decreased motility.— The full study—"Light Emitted from Media Devices at Night is Associated with Decline in Sperm Quality" (7) makes for fairly terrifying reading.

To learn more on this topic, I met one of the world's foremost sleep researchers and experts, Matthew Walker, at his Airbnb in London. And, surprisingly, he was tired.

Having been booked for an illustrious talk in front of thousands, he'd made an Airbnb reservation error. He'd found a place to stay online in London's Soho district. When he arrived, he discovered it was opposite the renowned classy establishment Tiger Tiger. It just so happens Tiger Tiger closes at 4am, at which point the noisy, boisterous patrons leave and proceed to wake up the locals. So, the world's top sleep guru was not particularly well rested.

But, boy, does he know a lot about sleep. He told me about a study of people who'd looked at an iPad before bed. It found that those who'd been in front of a screen had a 50% decrease in melatonin levels all night, as well as disrupted REM sleep. People also felt consistently "less refreshed" by their sleep, and this effect lasted for two to three days afterwards as well.

Then we talked about the solution, which is the color amber. You want to create amber "campfire light" around the house. It's scientifically proven to increase your melatonin production (8) as you aren't looking at that harmful bright blue light. To do this, you can try the following:

■ Dim the lights around the house in the evening

- Use amber 'blue-blocking glasses' which block out bright light.

- Have amber USB nightlights in the bedroom for a calming evening glow

- Use F:Lux on your computer screen if you are using it late. This syncs with the sun's position wherever you are in the world to reduce the blue in your screen as it gets dark outside.

I do all of this every night until lights out, and then ensure I sleep in a room that is as dark as possible. The glasses are particularly effective. Unfortunately blue-blocking glasses make you look like a lab technician. That is an interesting look on a night out, so I tend to only wear them at home.

BLUE-BLOCKING GLASSES TIP

Amber glasses are amazing for winding down at night. If you are feeling brave, feel free to wear them out on the town or in the pub with friends. But you mustn't wear them while driving. They completely cut the color blue out of your vision. That means you can't see a flashing blue light from the emergency services.

There is one further stage that might help you take your sleep to the next level. It is a $1.79 (£1.20) hack that will change your evenings. It does require craft skills, but don't worry: I'm not going all *Blue Peter* on you (attention American readers: this is a niche UK kids TV reference). If we are serious about blocking the blue light in our homes in the evening, we want to be looking at the devices that create that light. With a simple purchase that cost me almost nothing and some adhesive putty, I've managed to block the blue light on my Kindle, alarm clock, and even certain lights around the home which I only use at night. Without further ado, here is my $1.79 hack that will change your bedroom:

■ Buy an amber transparent sheet

■ Cut to size around your Kindle, alarm clock, and any other bedroom devices.

■ Blue light successfully blocked.

This worked so well, I then turned my attention to the kitchen. For the lights there, I went to a specialist stage lighting company and bought an amber light gel sheet that can withstand high temperatures. This is still very cheap.

It's surprising how relaxing this new lighting is. Although it does make our house look like the red light district.

Campfire light is your friend in the evening. You'll feel so much calmer and more ready for bed once you create it. It'll make you sleep better. And if you must watch Netflix in bed, get those glasses on and fire up F:Lux.

OPTIMIZE YOUR DEVICES FOR SLEEP: TOTAL RED MODE

There is a "Night Shift" mode on the iPhone (Android has a similar option) which makes the phone a warmer hue once it gets dark outside. Even at full strength, however, it's still quite bright.

So here's an effective workaround to completely cut all the blue light from your phone. This is a good hack to make the iPhone screen totally red at night. It will help you create more melatonin in the evenings pre-bedtime. That'll make you sleep better and deeper.

■ Pick up your iPhone and head to Settings

■ Then go to Accessibility > Display & Text Size > Color Filters. Switch this on and select Color Tint. Turn the Intensity and Hue dials all the way to the right, then switch off Color Filters again.

■ Then go back to Accessibility > Accessibility Shortcut and select Color Filters so there is a tick alongside that option.

■ Triple click your home button. Your screen will now be red. Triple click it again and the red switches off.

You now have a totally blue-blocked phone to help you wind down for sleep in the evening and power you up the next day.

This genuinely helps me wind down after dark. There is an easy test I have tried to confirm how effective this is. One night when it was late and I was looking at my totally red screen, I made the mistake of triple clicking the home button so I came out of Total Red Mode. The screen was surprisingly, and unpleasantly bright on my eyes. I don't want to do that again.

When the sun goes down, triple click to make your screen red and notice if you start to sleep better soon afterward.

YOUR SLEEP SANCTUARY: DESIGNING THE IDEAL BEDROOM FOR SLEEP

There are two good reasons for optimizing and upgrading those eight magical hours of slumber. You'll sleep better *and* have more bounce the next day.

Let's start with your bed. You know that "new car smell". That's off-gassing, and while some people might like the smell, it's not something you want to breathe in. Off-gassing is the release of chemicals (VOCs) from new products like cars, sofas, and items found in the bedroom too.

VOCs can include including benzene, acetaldehyde and formaldehyde. You don't need a degree in chemistry to know you probably want to swerve inhaling those. Researchers at the American Chemical Society have found that this is particularly important for young children as the mattresses warm up at night while being slept on: though they did emphasize the need for more studies (9). VOCs can irritate the eyes, nose and throat, and over-exposure to VOCs has been linked to cancer (10).

Optimize Your Mattress

These are all good reasons to focus on cleaning up our bedroom environment, specifically our mattress and pillow. Invest in an organic mattress. It'll make you feel good, although a little bit poorer—organic mattresses aren't particularly cheap.

I sleep on an Una Mattress. There's nothing nasty in it—certified organic materials from the groves of Hevea trees, no smelly petrochemicals, and no fire-retardant chemicals. I only started noticing just how good it is once I slept on a hotel bed. Boy, does the back hurt after a night elsewhere, compared to my lovely home mattress. I have no idea if that's off-gassing or something else, but it definitely gave me mattress meh.

There is one downside to my organic mattress. It is the heaviest bed I have ever known. It's a little impractical for moving house, or even moving room... but worth it for such a good night's sleep.

Optimize Your Duvet

Is it time to get a bit more selfish about sleep? After all, we do it for a third of our lives and we can't share it. So, how can we get the environment just right?

Again, go organic and natural to avoid any nasties. Hypoallergenic wool can be a good option. And then consider going radical. Perhaps "one bed, two duvets" is the answer? This is a Scandinavian sleep tradition that also is popular in Germany and Austria: it means your other half isn't kept awake by your shuffling around to get comfy. You get to choose your own personal temperature control and blanket weight, and you are less likely to be disturbed by your partner.

It all adds up to an unconventional bedroom, in many other Western cultures, but happy sleepers. As a Norwegian follower of mine said to me after I started looking into this:

"Seriously? One duvet? We'd be divorced. A duvet each is the way to go!"

It' s all in the name of sleeping better, and feeling livelier and healthier the next day.

RECHARGE WHILE YOU SLEEP

Your brain can only consciously think of a few things at once. That means it has a massive "hard drive". There is a concept in NLP called the "unconscious mind", which deals with all the things on the hard drive that just whir away in the background. It is already working away while we sleep (hence our dreams) and we can give it a little nudge in the right direction.

- Before you drop off, ask your "unconscious mind" to think about three instances in the next 24 hours where you can take action to recharge or re-energize. Talk to yourself. It'll feel unnatural but that's okay.

- Go to sleep. Allow your mind's hard drive to work away in the background

- As the days and weeks pass, notice if you start to instinctively take more action to boost your energy. You might even start to feel more energized in your dreams too.

Admittedly, this method requires a small leap of faith. It is a bit unconventional to talk to yourself in this way. But it is useful. It works away behind the scenes while you sleep to recover your energy.

SLEEP AND TRAVEL: MORE JET, LESS LAG

Decent sleep on the go is particularly elusive. When I travel long distances, I suffer from pretty spectacular jet lag meh. Once at my destination, I'll find myself so tired by mid-afternoon that matchsticks couldn't keep my eyes propped open. And, at an obscenely early hour, I'll be awake but tired, chugging down coffee. That means I stay in the same vicious lagged-up cycle for days on end.

For a recent trip, I vowed to avoid this push/pull process entirely and enlisted the help of a piece of health tech with the best name in the business: *The Human Charger.*

It operates on the now-familiar premise that bright light stimulates our circadian rhythm. The unusual part is that the device shines light into your *ears*. The makers claim it is the only non-pharmaceutical intervention that is scientifically proven to help beat jet lag.

The timing couldn't have been better—I had a flight coming up from London to Puerto Rico. The time difference is four hours, so clearly more manageable than some flights, but ideal for a trial run.

Two days before flight: I download the *Human Charger* app and put in my flight details. It directs me to put the earbuds in my ear in the mornings on the days leading up to my flight. I sit there shining light into my ears for 12 minutes. I feel a gentle extra buzz and a little more get-up-and-go afterwards.

On the morning of the flight: Passport, check. Tickets, check. *Human Charger*, check. Ready. But the big question is still to be answered: can the Human Charger really help get rid of that sluggish, post-flight hangover feeling?

On the flight itself: my fellow passengers look on suspiciously as I insert bright lights into my ears on the flight as directed by the app. It tells me that bright light in the evening of my destination in Puerto Rico (late night back in London) will have an effect in keeping me up and alert and full of zest. If only the app would explain to the woman next to me that I'm not a member of an unearthly cult that likes to shine intense light in my ears. I'll be using it four separate times today, twice on the flight and twice after landing, for 12 minutes each session.

On the evening of the flight: Once I arrived in the Puerto Rican capital San Juan, the practicalities of using the device become tricky. I'm feeling awake, which is good, and I'm out on the town having fun with friends. But the pesky app keeps bugging me, wanting me to stick my headphones on. I skip a session. Whoops. But wow, it still seems to work. I've done three of my four sessions, and miraculously, I stay out until 2am (6am UK time). And I don't feel like a zombie.

One day after the flight: I wake early, annoyingly early in fact. This nifty gadget may have had me up late last night, but it doesn't seem to have affected the early starts that jet lag often brings. Undeterred, I use it again as directed that evening and sure enough I stay out late once again.

Two days after the flight: Once again, I wake earlier than I'd ideally like. This thing doesn't seem to help me fully adjust my sleep schedule to my new time zone, but there's no doubt I've felt plenty of extra evening oomph since I've been here.

Verdict: I definitely got a little buzz from *Human Charger*. I was able to stay out late right from the start of my holiday. The downsides are that you have to remember to keep putting on the light-emitting headphones, which I found surprisingly inconvenient, even with the phone reminders. You also look a little strange wearing it—not necessarily a hip look if you are in a meeting, out on the town or, really, doing anything other than spending time on your own. Overall, though, the *Human Charger* is definitely worth a go next time you take a flight.

ERGONOMIC NECK PILLOWS: COMFY TRAVEL SLEEPING

One more travel story: I recently embarked on an enjoyable walking adventure called The Three Peaks Challenge with 12 friends. It involved hiking up the highest peaks in Wales, England, and Scotland and doing the whole thing within 24 hours. As well as a lot of trekking in the dark, the Three Peaks small print doesn't advise you on the lack of sleep involved. In fact, it's quite the challenge to get any at all in a tiny minibus with no legroom and 12 other sweaty, snoring blokes.

I enlisted the help of a neck support travel pillow. It is scientifically proven to hold your neck in the right place. It props you up in an ergonomic position during rest, and it is light (weighing only 148 grams). You can simply fold it away in your bag afterwards, which helped in the bus as space was at a premium. The one I used was a Trtl Pillow.

It couldn't create more legroom in that minibus or stop my 12 friends snoring away as we bumped along the M6 north to Ben Nevis. But it did support my neck and allowed me to grab a few precious moments of sleep. Next time you need to hack a nap on the go, do check this one out.

To conclude this part of the book, sleep is one of most important areas in which to quantify improvements. As you start to realign your circadian rhythm and tap into your natural sleep rhythms, you will want to know which tweaks actually work for you and which ones can be discarded.

Remember that core NLP principle, "Do What Works". Remember to track your progress in the MEH-TRICS section of the book, with the help of a sleep tracker of some sort. This is where the simple, effective sleep trackers we've covered there will come in handy. There are some worthwhile free options too. The more you can measure what works, the more you'll be able to replicate that outstanding night's sleep again and again, and you might not realize just how much a particular tweak is working until you see the data.

References

1. Entrainment of the Human Circadian Clock to the Natural Light-Dark Cycle—https://www.cell.com/current-biology/comments/S0960-9822(13)00764-1

2. 2016 Global Mobile Consumer Survey: The market-creating power of mobile—https://www2.deloitte.com/content/dam/Deloitte/us/Documents/technology-media-telecommunications/us-global-mobile-consumer-survey-2016-executive-summary.pdf

3. Effects of light on human circadian rhythms, sleep and mood—https://www.ncbi.nlm.nih.gov/pmc/articles/PMC6751071/

4. Effects of Mobile Use on Subjective Sleep Quality—https://www.ncbi.nlm.nih.gov/pmc/articles/PMC7320888/

5. Blue light from light-emitting diodes elicits a dose-dependent suppression of melatonin in humans—https://journals.physiology.org/doi/full/10.1152/japplphysiol.01413.2009

6. Is Blue Light Bad For Your Health?—https://www.webmd.com/sleep-disorders/news/20170619/is-blue-light-bad-for-your-health

7. Light Emitted from Media Devices at Night is Associated with Decline in Sperm Quality—https://academic.oup.com/sleep/article-abstract/43/Supplement_1/A12/5847498?redirectedFrom=fulltext

8. The effects of blue-light filtration on sleep and work outcomes—https://doi.apa.org/record/2020-48711-001?doi=1

9. Mattresses could emit higher levels of VOCs during sleep—https://www.sciencedaily.com/releases/2019/07/190710103211.htm

10. Volatile Organic Compounds—https://www.lung.org/clean-air/at-home/indoor-air-pollutants/volatile-organic-compounds

Meh-busting Sleep Reminders...

1

Leave your phone out of the bedroom. Get longer, deeper sleep and banish sleep FOMO.

2

Avoid "blue light" in the evening. Use red and amber light filters to increase melatonin and REM sleep.

3

Enhance your sleep environment. Optimize your mattress and duvet. Do whatever it takes to improve your sleep.

Chapter Nine

Meh-trics

"

What's measured improves.

PETER DRUCKER

"

Why this theme?

This is where the magic happens. In this final section, we bring together everything we've learned in order to ensure you're choosing the methods that work best for you. We collect stats on HRV, sleep, diet, health, and even DNA to create our own unique energy template. Here's why.

There are numerous techniques in this book, and...

■ Some will give you an instant jolt.

■ Others will provide a slow, steady drip of extra vitality.

■ And some might not be effective for you. (I'm just being realistic here.)

So the real magic comes when you start tracking. You ask yourself: what works best? And then you know you should keep doing it.

Remember, what's measured improves, so let's look at the importance of tracking your progress.

What can you expect in this section?

I will encourage you to take one minute each evening to take your metrics. We will consider everything from a multitude of different apps, sites, forms, spreadsheets, and even a little black book in which make a few notes on your day. You can simply work out your preferred way of collecting metrics.

These stats will end up being the basis for your own personal energy template. And don't worry, the process of collecting these metrics always takes one minute or less a day.

Each evening we will ask; what were the methods that supercharged your energy? What gave you a boost in a low moment? What methods reliably gave you a quick lift? And did anything not work so well?

Then, anytime you need more zest in the future, you can analyze your metrics. We'll look at how to do that too. Next time you aren't sure if something has been effective or not, you will have the data there to prove what works. You will have collected your own energy evidence. Bye, bye guesswork.

WHAT METRICS TO COLLECT: THE CROISSANTS MIGHT HAVE TO GO

You can collect data points on everything from sleep, diet, heart health, and exercise to just about anything else you can think of. So what should you collect metrics on?

I encourage you to get creative. For instance, if you suspect that every time you eat a croissant you have a 20% energy slump, you might want to track your croissant consumption. If the metrics prove a link between croissants and meh moments, you can then make a decision on whether the croissants will have to go. We are aiming for a level of personalized detail that will reveal hidden but important energy boosts.

Potential areas to track

- Energy levels
- Happiness
- Focus

- Workout length and quality
- Length of sleep
- Quality of sleep
- What time you went to bed
- Heart rate
- Heart rate variability
- Food eaten
- Calories
- Carbs
- Time of meals
- Exercise
- Supplements taken
- Any of the techniques in this book
- Croissant consumption (or any similar foodstuff)

For the subjective areas above such as energy levels or happiness levels, I suggest marking yourself with a number out of 10. You could also use a percentage.

I am an unashamed nerd when it comes to tracking stuff. It has to take less than 60 seconds at night though, because who wants to spend hours doing this stuff? I track anything and everything—lifestyle factors, supplements, energy levels and sleep quality, plus anything else I'm focusing on.

There really is no limit to what you might track. Years ago, I realized I was suffering stomach problems after eating nuts. But not all nuts. So I collected some nut metrics. That's a sentence I never thought I'd utter in public. A month later I'd uncovered the culprit—cashew nuts were making me bloated. Other nuts were no problem. Who knew? Certainly not me. I'd spent years feeling rubbish after eating cashews, but never realized it until I measured it. Nowadays I avoid the evil cashew nut like the plague. And my gut is much happier for it.

So pick a few areas to track. As you go through the book, add anything that you think might be having a big positive (or negative) impact.

Here is the process..

1. Take one minute a day to compile your energy metrics (more information on this to follow.)

2. After a while, look at the data and see what's working best. If, on the days you exercise, you are shown to be having a significant increase in energy levels, that is useful data.

3. Next time you need a boost, you have a proven routine to follow. You can't argue with the metrics.

Now let's look at the ways you can collect your data. Choose whatever works for you.

ONLINE FORMS: HAPPY COWS GIVE GOOD MILK

There are scientific studies that show that happy cows make better milk. One even found that, when farmers give cows a name and treat them as an individual, they can increase their annual milk yield by almost 500 pints (1).

Being happy is clearly good for cows, so I decided to collect some metrics to see if I could make myself a "happy cow". In this instance I used a good old-fashioned spreadsheet. Using Google Forms and Google Sheets, I tracked how much fun I had had on any particular day. I measured this by giving myself a "fun" score out of 10. The more fun activities in my day, the higher the score.

The results were spectacular. When there was very little "fun" on a particular day (below 5/10), my daily energy level was down 21.6%. A huge change. For me, lifestyle improvements are the quickest way to living with more vitality, and when I collect some data on it, I have proof of which changes work.

Conclusion: happy cows make better milk, and happy humans make more energy.

The Google Form is possibly my favorite way to collate the data in one place. It sends it to Google Sheets, where you can easily run some analysis. If you're interested in setting this up for yourself, I've recorded a special video step-by-step guide over on my website. It'll make it super easy for you. Head to www.tonywrighton.com/meh-xtras to get this and other bonuses.

If spreadsheets don't appeal, there are various other methods I use to track my progress.

USE AN APP: THERE ARE A MILLION DIFFERENT APPS FOR THAT. OKAY, EIGHT AT LEAST

Apps are sometimes even easier than a form to fill out at night. Your 60 seconds might become 30. Some of them provide meh-tric analysis too. If you'd rather use an app, there are a number that can help us track our meh levels. These apps are all free or affordable: there are links in the Meh Directory.

- *Optimized*, *Track This For Me*, and *Heads Up Health* focus on generalized tracking of whatever you want.

- *Daylio* works well because it's so simple. It takes seconds to fill out every evening, and is a fully customizable tracking app based on mood. They say it can help to "create some useful habits like running, eating more healthy or waking up earlier."

■ *Yolife* helps you get insights into the most important health areas of your life and an estimation of how long you will live in good health. This is all apparently based on scientific studies.

■ *Cara* focuses on digestion. It's not perfect, but could be handy if you suffer from IBS or other similar issues.

■ *Exist* and *Gyroscope* analyze your metrics and look for correlations, which is helpful. The subscription on these two services costs more though, and I find the Google form version above works as well.

■ There are a couple of excellent free sleep tracking apps that can help you geek out on sleep stats—*Sleep Cycle* and *Sleep Space*.

TOTALLY USELESS BUT QUITE INTERESTING

The app Sleep Cycle offers up all sorts of useless extra info, including the fact that people in Belgium are—at the time of writing—sleeping 15% better on average than people in Vietnam. And people in South Africa go to bed on average more than two hours earlier than people in Turkey. Is your bedtime routine more South African or Turkish?

USE A WEARABLE: IF IT'S GOOD ENOUGH FOR THE NBA AND UFC

Health wearables have become huge business. They are devices that are worn 24 hours a day which track various markers such as sleep quality, heart rate, heart rate variability (HRV), body temperature, exercise and an ever-growing list of what affordable technology can measure.

The concern with many wearable devices is they generate lots of data without being very helpful when it comes to the question of how to use it. Some say there's not much point in knowing your overnight respiratory rate, for example, if you aren't given insights as to what to do with that information.

So let's see if we can extrapolate some useful data out of wearables.

The Oura Ring is the "smart ring" made famous by the NBA, UFC, and Prince Harry. Sales exploded when Harry was spotted wearing one. I've been using it for years, but that didn't have the same public impact, naturally. It's a tracking device you wear on your finger. This little ring hit the headlines after research which suggested it can predict COVID-19 symptoms three days early (2). The NBA and UFC subsequently gave the ring to their players to track early COVID-19 symptoms. Oura also teamed up with the Red Bull Formula One Team to become the team's first ever "health technology partner".

DID YOU KNOW

Legendary UFC fighter Daniel Cormier is adamant that the Oura Ring helped him turn up for the final ever UFC fight in his long and illustrious career. It let him know he had a raised temperature, higher resting heart rate, and lower "recovery score".

Because of this information he was able to correctly identify he was suffering from COVID-19, self-isolate, and then recover properly for the fight.

More COVID-specific research needs to be done on this device: however, its other insights are also interesting. You might learn all sorts of things. For instance, it can correctly identify when I have had a couple of glasses of wine. I've consistently found that after small amounts of red wine, white wine or prosecco, my HRV scores are way down. My resting heart rate increases and my deep sleep drops off the chart. This tells me that fizz at night means a lack of fizz the next day. Where the tracking is particularly useful, though, is that the same thing doesn't happen if I drink other alcohols like rum.

You might start to see how wearables can help you measure your meh, then change it. Of course, the beauty of tracking is that you will develop your own personal insights. As an example of how you can use the information from a good wearable, here are a couple ways they've helped me manage my meh:

1. Meditation before bed seems to have a beneficial effect on my sleeping heart rate and HRV. Just ten minutes seems to do the trick.

2. Consistent good exercise and workouts seems to bring my heart rate down. Sitting around doing nothing seems to raise my heart rate.

One more important point. You want a wearable that has an airplane mode. Not all trackers have this feature. It means minimal EMFs on your body while you sleep/wear your device. Apple Watch provides airplane mode, as does Oura Ring. The Whoop Band is another option. Ideally the wearable won't have a screen, switches or flashing lights to distract you either.

If you don't want to invest in a fancy tracker there are some good free options. The options that can help you measure heart rate variability and heart rate are surprisingly accurate. You only need a cell phone, and you can get started on these in seconds.

The app *Instant Heart Rate* is a good starting point. It describes itself as the "most accurate mobile heart rate monitor", which means you can take your heart rate any time. This app helped me realize that double cream on my strawberries was giving me a serious histamine reaction. It was spiking my heart rate up to 120bpm. Which is a shame, as I rather like double cream.

The app *HRV4Training* allows you to track your HRV daily and follow your parasympathetic nervous system activity over time, providing some great stats. You just put your finger over your smartphone camera lens every morning. Then it provides correlations, HRV changes and trends and some more specialist info for runners and cyclists.

These apps all fit the bill of providing personalized critical trend data that you help you measure and improve your moods and energy.

WRITING IT DOWN: WHAT GEORGE WASHINGTON AND IPHONES HAVE IN COMMON

The first US president was an enthusiastic—some might say obsessive—diary writer. He just loved writing in his diary. He wrote diary entries on all sorts of stuff: politics, war, travel and much more. He was apparently especially keen on writing diaries on farming conditions. These diaries mattered so much to him that once he went on a long trip and forgot his diary, and was deeply frustrated when he discovered he'd left it behind. So much so that he ordered a lackey to immediately jump on their horse to go and find it at his residence. "It will be found, I presume, on my writing table", he said. "Put it under a good strong paper cover, sealed up as a letter."

Why did he write so much down? He simply realized how important it is to "derive useful lessons from past errors". He planned for the future, and recorded what he did with his time so he could return to have a look at it and learn from it.

Nowadays you can keep a diary, a journal, an iPhone app, or use emails you send yourself. You could even save it in "Notes" on your phone. If iPhones, or smartphones, or laptops had been invented quite a lot earlier, perhaps George Washington would have written his stuff that way instead. (See, now you've worked out the tenuous title of this section.) Or perhaps he would have stuck to his trusty pen and paper either way.

I've kept diaries and notebooks of different kinds for years. As social psychologist James Pennebaker observed in the book *Opening up By Writing It Down*, there is a particular brain/body connection that gets activated through the physical process of writing things down.

GATHERING POSITIVITY METRICS: YOUR LITTLE BLACK BOOK

To achieve what we want, it's a good idea to point our mind in the right direction. We have to achieve lots of what one of my original NLP coaches, the sports mind coach Karl Morris, calls "little victories". And it is good to remind yourself of these victories as well as to learn from your mistakes.

Let's adapt a core NLP technique that will help us gather metrics, then immediately learn from them. Grab a piece of paper and write out three simple headings:

- Good
- Better
- How

In the "Good" column, write what went well today.
In the "Better" column, write what could have been better.
In the "How" column, write how it could have been better.

In this way, you are successfully connecting with the "little victories" in your day. You also powerfully reframe those events that didn't go so well so you can learn from them. Use this exercise daily with a particular focus on energy.

Up in my loft, I have numerous black Moleskine books full to the brim with my daily musings written out in this way. Sometimes I dig them out and learn something new all over again. Karl started encouraging me to do this almost ten years ago, He told me "you can always achieve something in the next 24 hours, and the sense of completion is very satisfying. It might take 15 years to achieve your big goal, but look at what you achieved today."

Karl has worked with numerous world-beating sports stars so he knows what he is talking about. However, as crap as your day might have been, this brief process helps to a) positively reframe it in the moment so you feel better; and b) maintain a sense of momentum by reminding yourself of your constant "little victories", which are all leading towards your bigger goal of having more energy.

As Washington would say, you then "profit from your dearly bought experience."

NEXT STEPS: DETAILED HEALTH TESTING

As we near the end of the book, let's think about the future and consider more advanced metrics. How much money would health providers save if they tested people when they were healthy, rather than waiting until they got sick? And how much healthier and more energized would our lives be? It feels like we are slowly waking up to the ways in which the current approach leaves it all a bit late. But don't expect to be offered a comprehensive annual sweep of preventive testing any time soon. You'll have to be proactive and organize this yourself.

More in depth health testing and tracking is a good idea. This applies if you have a health issue, but also if you have want to generally optimize your health and energy long into the future.

This is something that varies quite considerably by country, and it is nearly always best to start with the expert advice of your health practitioner. However, lots of people wonder about where to get testing done, and there are plenty of options. It often isn't cheap, so consider these tests as an investment in your future vitality.

Viome is a futuristic testing kit and app which tells you exactly what foods and supplements you should and shouldn't be consuming. It is available in the USA, UK and elsewhere.

Omnos analyzes your DNA, biomarkers and lifestyle to understand the biggest influences on your overall wellness. Omnos is a relatively new company, and the user experience so far is great. Their dashboard effectively takes you through the process of getting the right tests and then helps you to interpret the results (the key bit).

Genetic testing is available from the likes of *23andme, SelfDecode* and many more. It includes more than 55 health reports that meet FDA requirements, and you can then run the results through other results like *Strategene* or *Found My Fitness* for more information.

GENETIC TESTING: DO YOU HAVE THE MOSQUITO BITE GENE?

Do you have meh in your genes? And if so, what can you do about it?

Some people win the genetic lottery. Lucky them. Others of us are born with "meh genes". (Note, there is not actually an official gene named the meh gene. Yet.)

But even if they do, they still have to look after those genes, otherwise they will start to play up, and not work as well.

I was recently lucky enough to spend time with a world-famous neurological expert. He'd just made an exciting, controversial public statement:

"Virtually no one in the future should have to die from Alzheimer's."

Clearly a big claim, but if anyone has the credentials to back it up, Dr. Dale Bredesen does. His book on Alzheimer's went straight to the Number 1 spot on Amazon in every book category. Pretty impressive for a topic that is, let's face it, a bit of a tough sell. His sales briefly surpassed Hillary, Oprah, and any other bestselling authors known by only one name.

I love his work, because I am slightly more likely than average to develop Alzheimer's myself. I am a carrier of the APOE4 gene that makes this cruel disease more probably. I am one of the 25% of people with one copy of this gene. If you haven't got your genetic make-up tested yet with 23andMe or another company, then I guess this info might seem a little daunting. Admittedly, it's not exactly fun to find out that you are more likely to die from a neuro-disease than your next door neighbor.

There is reason for hope, though. You're going to think I'm strange now, but I consider it a blessing to have found out I have the Alzheimer's gene. Obviously, I don't want to suffer from it, and I have huge amounts of empathy and sympathy for anyone who does. But just having the information that it is more of a possibility for me has forced me to make changes to protect my energy. I watch my sleep, keep my brain working well and I've changed my diet. I eat a bit less meat, and focus more on fresh veggies. And I feel even better. That's not so bad, is it?

This area is known as epigenetics. It's the study of how your behavior, environment and lifestyle affect the expression of your genes.

Dr. Bredesen is one of the world's foremost experts on Alzheimer's. He's seen case upon case over many years of patients, who sometimes already experienced advanced neurological decline. Many do have the same gene I have. He has halted, and in some cases reversed their symptoms. He has a particular focus on exercise, diet, lifestyle changes and regular testing for various biomarkers: and those patients didn't have the advantage of having started on this course 30 years earlier. We do have to opportunity to do that. Epigenetics means we are in control of our own destiny.

A DNA test is normally just a spit test. Do it at home, whack it in the post, and a few weeks later you'll have all this information in front of you. Among other things you'll find out whether you have either one or two copies of the APOE4 gene. That's just one of thousands of genes covered by the testing.

You'll discover all sorts of things this way. Perhaps you'll have a copy of the gene that doesn't process coffee well, and then you'll know that drinking it earlier in the day is going to help you sleep better. Again, epigenetics helps you to start being more in control of your own destiny.

Or have you ever felt like you get bitten more by mosquitos than others? You're on holiday, you go out for dinner, and you come back covered in bites, while your family and friends seem to have been ignored? Actually, there is not one particular "mosquito bite gene" (though that would be a good name for one): instead there is a set of 285 genes that can be used to compile a Mosquito Bite Trait report, confirming that some people attract more mosquitoes and react more severely to bites.

I presume you are not reading this book to avoid getting bitten by mosquitos, although that would be nice. But there are other important indicators that are important for energy, health, and longevity, such as the BRCA1/BRCA2 "breast cancer" gene. This has been found to impact the chances of having certain types of cancers. Again, the idea of having this information is to help you live longer and more healthily. In this instance, that might involve testing more regularly with mammograms and breast MRIs, adapting your lifestyle and getting regular expert consultations.

Having this knowledge is probably not for everyone. I believe it to be empowering though, and the pace of progress in decoding our genetic make-up is astonishing. Healthcare is going to be totally different in 30 years time. It'll be based much more on your own personal genetic make-up. And you can start to be in control of your destiny right now.

ANALYZING RESULTS: YOUR ENERGY EVIDENCE

With metrics, we can learn daily what works best for us. I've found that the areas which have the biggest influence tend to show up almost straight away. You'll quickly spot correlations and interesting trends. If you want to get fancy, you can draw graphs or pie-charts. Google Sheets will analyze the data you collect and present trends to you, which is very helpful. Many of the apps listed above will do the same thing.

So here are my basics. These non-negotiables come from years of tracking what busts my own meh.

- Exercise
- Relaxing
- Spending way less time in front of screens
- Prioritizing having fun and being a "happy cow" (see earlier)

Then I start to go deeper with my metrics. On the days I exercise, relax, escape the screens and have lots of fun, I might get more creative. Or I might have a particular insight when I'm meditating. That's the power of knowing which things that energize me. What will yours be? What do you do when you have lots of energy, and how can you replicate it?

Remember, you are creating an effective, evidence-based personalized template for invigorating and enlivening your life when times get tough. You model your own excellence as you collect your energy evidence.

As you start to make changes, go easy on yourself. You won't get everything right all the time. The graph of your increasing energy levels will not be linear. Make small changes and commit to them. Don't aim too high at first. That may sound counter-intuitive in a book which is all about radically improving your energy levels, but for lasting change, it's best to start small. Author of the #1 NYT bestseller *Atomic Habits*, James Clear, says this:

"When you dream about making a change, excitement inevitably takes over and you end up trying to do too much too soon. The most effective way I know to counteract this tendency is to use the Two-Minute Rule, which states, "When you start a new habit, it should take less than two minutes to do."

Einstein once said, "Everything is energy,". He was right. Hopefully you are starting to understand the weird and wonderful ways in which your own personal vitality levels operate. I wish you the best of luck in boosting your energy and banishing your meh.

References

1. Happy cows produce more milk—https://www.scientistlive.com/content/happy-cows-produce-more-milk
2. WVU Rockefeller Neuroscience Institute and Oura Health unveil study to predict the outbreak of COVID-19 in healthcare professionals—https://wvutoday.wvu.edu/stories/2020/04/08/wvu-rockefeller-neuroscience-institute-and-oura-health-unveil-study-to-predict-the-outbreak-of-covid-19-in-healthcare-professional

Meh-busting Meh-trics Reminders...

1

Gather metrics. Use anything from a little black book to advanced apps. Track sleep, diet, lifestyle... anything that works.

2

Find correlations. Do more of what works. "Profit from your dearly bought experience".

3

Go next level. Learn from HRV, test key health biomarkers and investigate your DNA. All in the name of more energy.

Directory

Here is a list of many of the products, services, books and practices that I recommend and have used myself.

For my full up-to-date list with hyperlinks for easy use, discounts (in some cases quite large) and my latest favorite biohacks, visit www.tonywrighton.com/meh-xtras. You'll find the latest version there, along with other bonuses and reader extras.

- 23andme—genetic testing.

- 40 Years Of Zen— for the deepest possible dive into neurofeedback.

- Air Angel—an air purifier from HypoAir that kills 99 percent of allergens, odors, germs, and viruses, including various forms of coronavirus. It has been successfully tested on SARS-CoV-2 (the COVID-19 virus). I use it in my bedroom and office.

- Altra trainers"'zero drop" shoe, which means the sole is the same height as the toe and a little more padded, which nicely cushions my dodgy knees. Not quite as stylish as some but my favorite zero drop shoes.

- Berkey Water Filter—removes 99.9999999% of pathogenic bacteria and 99.999% of viruses while leaving the essential minerals your body needs.

- Binaural beats app—scientifically proven to induce altered states of consciousness such as more of an Alpha state (in which stress and anxiety are reduced—a proper chill-out zone), or a Gamma state (the ideas zone—for memory processing, language, learning).

- Blue-blocking glasses—there are lots of options but these are the ones I use.

- Blue-blocking USB booklight from Lencent—for reading at night.

- Bulletproof Charcoal—activated charcoal binds to toxins and helps get rid of them.

- Bulletproof Coffee Beans—low-toxin, low-mold organic coffee grown by reputable farmers.

- Bulletproof Cookbook—good low-carb recipes.

- CAR.O.L—your AI powered fitness bike. Get the same benefits of a 45-minute jog in two 20-second sprints on their bike.

- Dan Harris's 10% Happier app—a good meditation app.

- DAOfood Plus—a supplement that provides DAO, the primary enzyme that degrades ingested histamine. It also contains Vitamin C and Quercetin .

- Daylio—works well because it's so simple. It takes seconds to fill out every evening, and is a fully customizable tracking app based on mood. They say it can help "create some useful habits like running, eating more healthy or waking up earlier."

- Dr Hisham's mouth rinse—for "7 minutes of mouth joy'" How can you say no to that?

- Dr Hisham's Adult Vital Teeth Serum—posh toothpaste. It works.

- Dry Farms Wines—their natural wines are sugar-free, low-alcohol and low-sulfite.

- Evergreen coffee capsules—stainless steel capsules to put your coffee in, compatible with Nespresso®, Dolce Gusto® and others.

- EWG's Skin Deep site—search for all your personal care products and find out if they are safe.

- Exist—Track everything together. Understand your behavior.

- *Fast This Way*—an excellent book on everything to do with fasting from Dave Asprey.

- Flip-flops by Pluggz—containing "a proprietary carbon and rubber black plug embedded into the soles which allows for the free flow of electrons from the Earth into our bodies."

- F:Lux—a free download that warms up your computer display at night, to match your indoor lighting.

- Flourish—a breathwork app. Created by Richie Bostock. Apps like his have some great ideas for breathwork.

- Found My Fitness—analyzes DNA testing and lots of other great health resources.

- Freestyle Libre—Continuous Glucose Monitor (CGM) that lasts 14 days.

- Füm—an all-natural essential oil aromatherapy inhaler. Brilliant idea. For congestion, exercise, anxiety, and even nicotine cessation.

- Gadget Guard—a phone case snappily described as "the world's only case with patented technology proven to reduce cell phone radiation by up to 75% while maintaining signal strength".

- Get A Drip—pump in high strength Vitamin C and hydration. London-based.

- GlassesOff, eyesight app to naturally improve your vision.

- Glo—a website with a huge amount of workouts and meditations.

- Gyroscope—analyze your metrics and get insights.

- Ha'You Fit—where Qi Gong, fitness and breathwork meet.

- Hartig & Helling—an extremely low-radiation'baby monitor which works through a very low analogue radio signal.

- Higher Dose sauna blanket—an affordable infrared heat option.

- *Histamine Intolerance Cookbook* by Ketoko Guides (my company)—low histamine and mostly low-carb recipes

- Holden Qi Gong—Jump-Start Your Qi Gong Practice with Easy Online Classes.

- HRV4Training—this app allows you to track your HRV daily and follow your parasympathetic nervous system activity over time, providing some great stats.

- Human Charger—the makers claim it is the only non-pharmaceutical intervention that is scientifically proven to help beat jet lag.

- Instant Heart Rate—an app that claims to be the "most accurate mobile heart rate monitor".

- Instant Pot - a healthy, quick pressure cooker. It cooks, steams, sautés, makes (histamine intolerance friendly) yoghurts and so much more. So good I'm in danger of becoming an Instant Pot bore.

- James Nestor breath resources—excellent collection of breathwork videos in one place.

- Joovv—infrared light company so serious about what they do they've teamed up with the athletes of the San Francisco 49ers to help their recovery regime.

- Lambs—EMF-blocking underwear.

- LEMS shoes—wide shoes for my big paddle feet. Surprisingly stylish.

- Magnesium Breakthrough—for better sleep and looser joints.

- *Men Are From Mars, Women Are From Venus*—better relationships = less meh. The best-selling non-fiction hardback book of all time from the brilliant John Gray.

- Meriva—is a particularly bio-available form of curcumin/turmeric, which can help with the brain.

- Methylene Blue—can help with better memory, focus and mood and is proven safe at the given dosage level.

- Mindful Coffee—good organic coffee, with a nice buttery taste.

- Muse—"brain-sensing headband" which provides a surprising level of in-depth mind discovery.

- Night Shift mode—on the iPhone (Android has similar) which makes the phone a warmer hue in the evening.

- Oculus Quest 2—VR workouts are insanely enjoyable.

- Omnos—analyzes your DNA, biomarkers and lifestyle to understand the biggest influences on your overall wellness.

- Onegreenbottle—all stainless steel bottle with steel cap. Trust me, I went down this rabbit hole so you don't have to, not to mention investing in non-plastic cookware like silicon, iron, and stainless steel.

- Oura Ring—tracks sleep quality, heart rate, heart rate variability, body temperature, respiratory rate, exercise and lots more.

- P:volve—targeted Pilates-like workouts to improve your core

- Prolon—the 5-day fasting mimicking diet. Not for the faint-hearted.

- Readwise—syncs up with your Kindle highlights then sends you a daily email. You choose how many quotes you want a day.

- Resveratrol from Trans Health—for healthy aging. It helps the cardiovascular system, and protects against cancer and diabetes, with very little downside.

- SafeSleeve provides protection on your phone while you're holding it to your ear.

- Sam Harris's Waking Up app—for daily 10- or 20-minute meditation.

- Seeking Health Liposomal Glutathione—for energy, detox and wellness. Tastes like sewers but it gets the job done.

- Seeking Health Vitamin D—for immunity and health, especially in winter.

- SelfDecode—genetic testing and analysis.

- Sensate meditation pebble—hang it round your neck and it sends weird vibrations through your chest up into your head. It uses "the science of bone conduction" to send these vibrations up into your body.

- Sleep Cycle—a free sleep app. For an addictive geek out on sleep stats.

- Soleil Toujours—mineral sunscreen that doesn't make you look like a clown.

- Squatty Potty—for a more primal visit to the toilet.

- Standing desk—lots available. This is the one I use.

- Strategene—strategic genetic testing, also analyzes DNA and gene results.

- Sunlighten—low-EMF infrared sauna. Complete with Netflix screen.

- The 2-Meal Day, assistance on intermittent fasting.

- The Class—sweaty, genre-defying workouts that challenge mind and body.

- *The Complete Guide To Fasting*—Dr. Jason Fung and Jimmy Moore explain everything you ever wanted to know about fuel timings.

- The Histamine Intolerance Site—everything you need to know about histamine intolerance, plus a quiz and food list.

- The Wand—described as "A Wine Filter That Removes Histamines & Sulfite Preservatives".

- Theragun—an incredible percussive massage tool. Extraordinarily effective in easing away aches. Beware of cheap imitations as I can tell you from experience—they don't work.

- Think Dirty—an app that helps us discover potential toxins in household, personal care and beauty products.

- Tito's Handmade Vodka—micro-distilled six times in an old-fashioned pot.

- Trtl Pillow—a scientifically proven neck support travel pillow.

- Ullo—removes sulfites from wine. Helps alleviate your sore head the next day.

- Ugly—sparkling water with real fruit flavor, no additives or sweeteners.

- Una Mattress—certified organic materials from the groves of Hevea trees, no smelly petrochemicals, and no fire-retardant chemicals.

- Veristable—monitor your glucose levels, rediscover nutrition, find out what works for you. A seriously good product, but not cheap.

- Viome—is a futuristic testing kit and app tells you exactly what foods and supplements you should and shouldn't be consuming.

- Vivo Barefoot—perhaps the most stylish barefoot shoes.

- *Zero Waste Lifestyle*—excellent book for less clutter, more simplicity, helping the environment, getting more energy for the things that matter, and (a biggie) saving money.

What did you think?

Reviews are the absolute lifeblood of any book, and now I'd love your feedback. I wonder if you'd help me spread the word and write a 30-second review on Amazon. What did you love? What are the techniques that have suited you the best? What has busted your meh? Do tell me (and the world) all about it.

I intend to keep updating this guide based on the latest research and your feedback. It is a labor of love and I want to keep it relevant. I read all my reviews, so let me know what you think. Finally a big thank you from us all for your support.

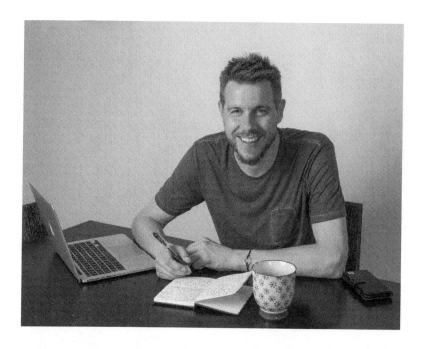

Made in the USA
Las Vegas, NV
14 April 2021